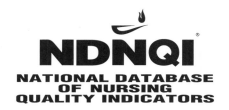

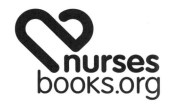

NDNQI Case Studies in Nursing Quality Improvement

Jennifer Duncan, PhD, RN

Isis Montalvo, MBA, MS, RN

Nancy Dunton, PhD

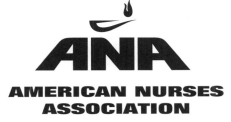

AMERICAN NURSES ASSOCIATION

SILVER SPRING, MARYLAND

2011

Library of Congress Cataloging-in-Publication Data

Duncan, Jennifer, RN.
    NDNQI case studies in nursing quality improvement / by Jennifer Duncan, Isis Montalvo, Nancy Dunton.
       p. ; cm.
    National Database of Nursing Quality Indicators case studies in nursing quality improvement
    Includes bibliographical references and index.
    ISBN-13: 978-1-55810-305-4 (pbk.)
    ISBN-10: 1-55810-305-8 (pbk.)
       1. Nursing—Standards—United States.   2. Nursing—Quality control—United States.   I. Montalvo, Isis.
II. Dunton, Nancy.   III. National Center for Nursing Quality (American Nurses Association)   IV. Title.
V. Title: National Database of Nursing Quality Indicators case studies in nursing quality improvement.
    [DNLM: 1. Nursing Care—standards—United States.   2. Quality Improvement—United States.
3. Databases as Topic—United States.   4. Hospitals—United States.   WY 100 AA1]
    RT85.5.D86   2011
    610.73—dc22

The opinions in this book reflect those of the authors and do not necessarily reflect positions or policies of the American Nurses Association. Furthermore, the information in this book should not be construed as legal or other professional advice.

Published by Nursesbooks.org
The Publishing Program of ANA
http://www.Nursesbooks.org

American Nurses Association
8515 Georgia Avenue, Suite 400
Silver Spring, MD 20910-3492
1-800-274-4ANA
http://www.Nursingworld.org/

Page design: Laura C. Johnson, VA
Cover design: AURAS Design, Silver Spring, MD
Typesetting: House of Equations, Inc., Arden, NC
Copyediting: Steven A. Jent, Denton, TX
Proofreading: Angela Forest, Wendy Moltrop (Editorial Experts, Inc; Columbia, MD)
Indexing: Gina Wiatrowski (Grammarians, Inc; Washington, DC)
Printing: Linemark Printing, Inc., Upper Marlboro, MD

Permission must be requested in writing from ANA to reuse or reprint any of the NDNQI benchmarks published in this book.

ISBN-13: 978-1-55810-305-4   SAN: 851-3481   2.5M   01/11
First printing: January 2011.

Contents

Contributors

About the Authors

Jennifer Duncan, PhD, RN
Research Associate, National Database of
Nursing Quality Indicators
University of Kansas School of Nursing

Jennifer Duncan is a writer and researcher for the National Database of Nursing Quality Indicators® (NDNQI®). Most recently, Dr. Duncan created an interactive online tutorial to help NDNQI members interpret their nursing-sensitive indicators and engage in quality improvement. Dr. Duncan was lead author of the acuity and risk adjustment study plan for NDNQI's Methods Development Team and co-author of the keynote address at NDNQI's 2010 conference. As an oncology nurse, she practiced at Memorial Sloan-Kettering Cancer Center and oncology clinics in Kentucky and Kansas. In 2007, Dr. Duncan received her PhD in nursing from the University of Kansas. She has published in *Cancer Nursing* and *Research in Nursing and Health* and is a member of the Sigma Theta Tau International Honor Society and the American Nurses Association.

Isis Montalvo, MBA, MS, RN
Director, National Center for Nursing Quality
American Nurses Association

Isis Montalvo directs and coordinates the interpretation and response to issues related to nursing quality and provides strategic direction and oversight to the National Center for Nursing Quality® (NCNQ®) and its database, the National Database of Nursing Quality Indicators® (NDNQI®), in which over 1,700 hospitals currently participate. She co-chairs the NDNQI Research Council and chairs the annual NDNQI Conference planning.

Ms. Montalvo has over 23 years experience in multiple areas of clinical and administrative practice with a focus on critical care and performance improvement. As a former NDNQI Site Coordinator, Quality Specialist, and Nursing Research Chair at a large urban facility, she brings expertise in data analysis, performance improvement, and nursing care evaluation. She has published articles and books on nursing quality improvement. In 1996, she received her Master's in Business Administration from the University of Baltimore in Maryland and her Master's of Science in Nursing Administration from the University of Maryland. She is a Critical Care Registered Nurse (CCRN) Alumnus and a member of multiple associations, and Phi Kappa Phi and Sigma Theta Tau Honor Societies.

Nancy E. Dunton, PhD
Research Professor,
School of Nursing
University of Kansas Medical Center

Nancy Dunton, with a joint appointment in the School of Medicine's Department of Health Policy and Management, has been the principal investigator for the National Database of Nursing Quality Indicators® (NDNQI®) since its inception in 1998. Under her direction, NDNQI has developed 19 nursing-sensitive indicators for acute care settings, four of which have been endorsed as national consensus standards by the National Quality Forum. Dr. Dunton has made numerous presentations and publications on NDNQI. She has served on panels for the National Quality Forum, the Agency for Healthcare Research and Quality, and the Joint Commission. Dr. Dunton received her PhD in Sociology from the University of Wisconsin.

Acknowledgments

The authors would like to thank the staff nurses and nursing leaders who make the daily difference in patient outcomes; the case study authors for sharing their stories so others may benefit from their knowledge and experience; Jianghua He, PhD, Brandon Crosser, MA, and the NDNQI® staff who identified hospitals with improved indicators and created the case study graphics; Marsha Russell for her administrative assistance with this project; and Rosanne Roe, Eric Wurzbacher, and the staff of Nursesbooks.org, the publishing program of ANA.

About the American Nurses Association

The American Nurses Association (ANA) is the only full-service professional organization representing the interests of the nation's 3.1 million registered nurses through its constituent member nurses associations and its organizational affiliates. The ANA advances the nursing profession by fostering high standards of nursing practice, promoting the economic and general welfare of nurses in the workplace, projecting a positive and realistic view of nursing, and lobbying the Congress and regulatory agencies on healthcare issues affecting nurses and the public.

About the National Center for Nursing Quality

The National Center for Nursing Quality® (NCNQ®) was created by ANA to address patient safety and quality in nursing care and nurses' work lives. The center advocates for nursing quality through research and measurement, advocacy in the national quality enterprise, collaborative learning, and consultative services. It also promotes the Nursing Quality Network. Issues such as the nursing workforce and impact on patient outcomes are tackled through innovative initiatives, which include the National Database of Nursing Quality Indicators® and Safe Staffing Saves Lives.

About Nursesbooks.org, The Publishing Program of ANA

Nursesbooks.org publishes books on ANA core issues and programs, including ethics, leadership, quality, specialty practice, advanced practice, and the profession's enduring legacy. Best known for the foundational documents of the profession on ethics, scope and standards of practice, and social policy, Nursesbooks.org is the publisher for the professional, career-oriented nurse, reaching and serving nurse educators, administrators, managers, and researchers, as well as staff nurses in the course of their professional development.

Chapter 1.
Evaluating and Improving Nursing Quality

Nurses have always been instrumental in improving patient safety and the quality of health care. As the nursing profession was born, Florence Nightingale used data she collected from her practice to convince the leaders of her day that sanitation improved survival rates. Today, bedside nurses and nursing leaders use data from the National Database of Nursing Quality Indicators® (NDNQI®) to help them keep patients safe and improve their nursing practice. This book provides an overview of nursing quality measurement and improvement methods, a step-by-step guide to using NDNQI data for quality improvement, and case studies of successful improvement initiatives in 11 U.S. hospitals.

Over the past 15 years, the mandate for improved quality of care has spread through all aspects of the healthcare system. The Institute of Medicine (IOM) defines quality of care as "the degree to which health services for individuals and populations increase the likelihood of desired health outcomes and are consistent with current professional knowledge" (2001). Landmark reports such as IOM's *To Err is Human* and *Crossing the Quality Chasm* brought attention to the many undesirable outcomes experienced by patients and the gap between scientific knowledge and clinical practice (IOM, 2000; 2001). Standardized measures of quality created by pioneers such as the American Nurses Association (ANA) have enabled nurses to begin closing the gap and improving outcomes.

Measures of quality (i.e., quality indicators) have made hospitals increasingly accountable for the nursing care they provide. Government and private insurers now use quality indicators for setting reimbursement rates. In particular, initiatives from the Centers for Medicare and Medicaid Services (CMS) have promoted the reporting and improvement of quality indicators. CMS's initiatives evolved from public reporting (no incentive offered) to pay-for-reporting (incentive for reporting measure) to pay-for-performance (payment or non-payment based on measure performance). The latter initiative holds healthcare organizations accountable for their quality of care by directly tying reimbursement to performance on standardized measures. Thus, nurses' work to improve patient safety has a greater financial impact than ever before, giving further value and importance to the profession and to individual nurses.

Multiple indicators are now used to evaluate the quality of nursing care. Each indicator measures one aspect of quality, such as the rate of hospital-acquired infections. To obtain a thorough view of quality, multiple indicators are needed. When an indicator is a direct measure of nursing or is strongly influenced by the care that nurses provide, it is called a *nursing-sensitive indicator*. Many hospitals report their performance on nursing-sensitive indicators to NDNQI.

National Database of Nursing Quality Indicators

NDNQI is the national leader in nursing quality measurement. As of July 2010, 16,579 nursing units in 1,540 hospitals submitted data on nursing-sensitive indicators such as pressure ulcers, patient falls, healthcare-associated infections, number and qualifications of nurses, and more. Every three months, participating nursing units download comparative data reports generated by NDNQI analysts. Reports promote quality improvement by enabling each unit to compare its staffing levels, nursing practices, and patient outcomes to similar units in similar hospitals. For instance, the quarterly report for a critical care unit in a teaching hospital might reveal its pressure ulcer rate to be above the 75th percentile for critical care units in teaching hospitals nationally. Such a report is intended to trigger a quality improvement effort aimed at lowering pressure ulcer occurrence on that unit.

NDNQI was created as part of ANA's Patient Safety and Quality Initiative to identify the linkages between staffing and patient outcomes. During the mid-1990s, extensive reviews of published evidence and pilot testing by seven state nurses associations led to the definition of reliable and valid nursing quality indicators (Montalvo, 2007). In 1998, ANA established the National Center for Nursing Quality (NCNQ®) and its measurement database, the National Database of Nursing Quality Indicators. The NCNQ advocates for nursing quality and patient safety through research and measurement, collaborative learning, and engagement in the national quality enterprise. The database was originally managed by the Midwest Research Institute and the University of Kansas (KU) School of Nursing under contract to ANA; NDNQI became managed solely by the KU School of Nursing in 2001. When first established, the database consisted of 30 hospitals reporting data on four newly-defined indicators.

Since that time, the database has continually grown in size and content. Hospitals from all 50 states and the District of Columbia now participate in NDNQI, along with seven international hospitals. Virtually all types of hospitals are represented. As of July 2010, 821 non-teaching hospitals, 550 teaching hospitals, and 169 academic medical centers participate in quarterly data reporting. Behavioral health, rehabilitation, oncology, pediatrics, cardiology, and women's specialty hospitals are included in NDNQI, along with 1,344 general hospitals whose bed sizes range from under 50 to over 900. The American Nurses Credentialing Center (ANCC) has awarded 368 NDNQI-member hospitals (24% of the total in the database) Magnet® recognition for excellence in nursing services. Currently, over 1,700 hospitals participate in NDNQI.

As participation has grown, so have the comparison group options available in NDNQI reports. Nursing units may view comparison data grouped by teaching status, hospital bed size, geographic location (state, census division, and metropolitan status), hospital specialty, unit specialty, Magnet recognition status, or Medicare case mix index category. Comparative reports are also available for multi-hospital health systems. Regardless of comparison group, all reports are stratified by unit type (e.g., adult surgical units are compared to other adult surgical units; pediatric intensive care units [ICUs] are compared to other pediatric ICUs). The combination of unit-level data with a wide selection of comparison groups allows nursing units to draw meaningful conclusions about their performance.

NDNQI collects quarterly data on nurse staffing and patient care indicators and also conducts an annual survey of RNs to evaluate job satisfaction and the nursing work environment. Many indicators collected by NDNQI are endorsed by the National Quality Forum (NQF), a non-profit organization that promotes standardized measures of healthcare quality. Four of the original indicators developed by ANA were selected for NQF's Nursing-Sensitive Care Performance Measure Set: nursing care hours per patient day, skill mix, patient falls, and falls with injury (NQF, 2004, 2009). NDNQI has incorporated additional NQF-endorsed measures in their data collection, including pressure ulcer prevalence, restraint prevalence, healthcare-associated infections, voluntary nurse turnover, and the Practice Environment Scale. Appendix A lists the quality indicators currently collected by NDNQI. NDNQI continually works to ensure the reliability and validity of their indicators through annual reliability studies of individual indicators and ongoing participant training to promote compliance with precise data collection and entry protocols. Reliable and valid indicators enable public reporting of nursing quality data.

Hospitals that participate in NDNQI benefit substantially from measuring their nursing quality. Benchmarking to peers can spur quality improvement initiatives that reduce costly adverse events and enhance the hospital's reputation. Additionally, CMS now stipulates participation in a systematic clinical database registry for nursing-sensitive care as one of the criteria for receiving full Medicare reimbursement rates. Hospitals that do not participate in NDNQI or another qualifying database will experience a 2% reduction in the annual inflation update to Medicare payment rates (CMS, 2010). Participation in NDNQI also fulfills the nursing-sensitive data collection requirements for hospitals seeking to obtain or retain Magnet recognition for nursing excellence.

NDNQI continually strives to enhance the usefulness of nursing quality indicators. Interactive self-paced online training helps nurses use their NDNQI comparative reports for quality improvement. Researchers at NDNQI are investigating statistical adjustment techniques that would allow mixed acuity units to compare their staffing and patient outcomes to peers. NDNQI's annual conferences highlight examples of successful quality improvement and promote diffusion of innovations in nursing. With diverse and growing participation, widely accepted indicators, and ongoing development projects, NDNQI is well poised to lead nursing quality measurement in the twenty-first century.

Structure, Process, and Outcomes in Nursing Quality

Comprehensive evaluation of nursing care requires three types of indicators: structure, process, and outcome. Quality theorist Avedis Donabedian (1966, 2003) introduced structure, process, and outcome as distinct yet related approaches to measuring healthcare quality. Using all three gives a complete, balanced view of nursing care. *Importantly, the structure of nursing care influences the processes of care, and both affect outcomes* (Montalvo & Dunton, 2007). Figure 1 provides an example of the relationship between a few of the structure, process, and outcome indicators collected by NDNQI.

Structure refers to the environment in which care is provided. Structure encompasses the number and

qualifications of staff, availability of equipment and supplies, and the nursing work environment (e.g., participation in hospital policy making, supportive leadership, staffing adequacy, and collegial nurse–physician interaction). Structure would also include such factors as staff specialty certification, retention and turnover, health information technology (e.g., electronic health records and hand-held devices with nursing applications software, computerized physician order entry, barcode-assisted medication administration), and hospital characteristics (e.g., teaching status, Magnet recognition). *Structure sets the stage for quality by facilitating or limiting nurses' ability to provide care.* Donabedian (2003) views structure as the main determinant of the average quality of care a facility can offer. NDNQI structure measures (e.g., nursing hours per patient day, percent of hours supplied by RNs) help healthcare professionals and consumers evaluate how well equipped a unit is to offer quality nursing care.

Process refers to the activities of daily patient care. Assessment, care planning, medication administration, preventive interventions, evidence-based procedures, patient and family education, and nurse–patient interactions are all processes of care. *Processes are the things nurses do, or fail to do, that shape patient outcomes.* Processes that are known to contribute to desirable outcomes are an indication of quality care (Donabedian, 2003). Examples of process measures collected by NDNQI include the average number of pain assessments per pediatric patient in 24 hours and the percent of patients at risk for pressure ulcers who received preventive interventions.

Outcomes are changes in patients' health attributable to their care. Nursing-sensitive patient outcomes such as hospital- and unit-acquired pressure ulcers, falls, device-associated infections, and peripheral IV infiltrations are changes in patients' well-being that are influenced by the structure and process of nursing care. Outcomes are often viewed as the ideal approach to measuring quality. However, variations in patient characteristics (i.e., case mix) often interact with the processes of care to determine outcomes (Donabedian, 2003). For example, a critical care unit with immobile patients might not

FIGURE 1.
Example of Relationship Between Structure, Process, and Outcome Indicators

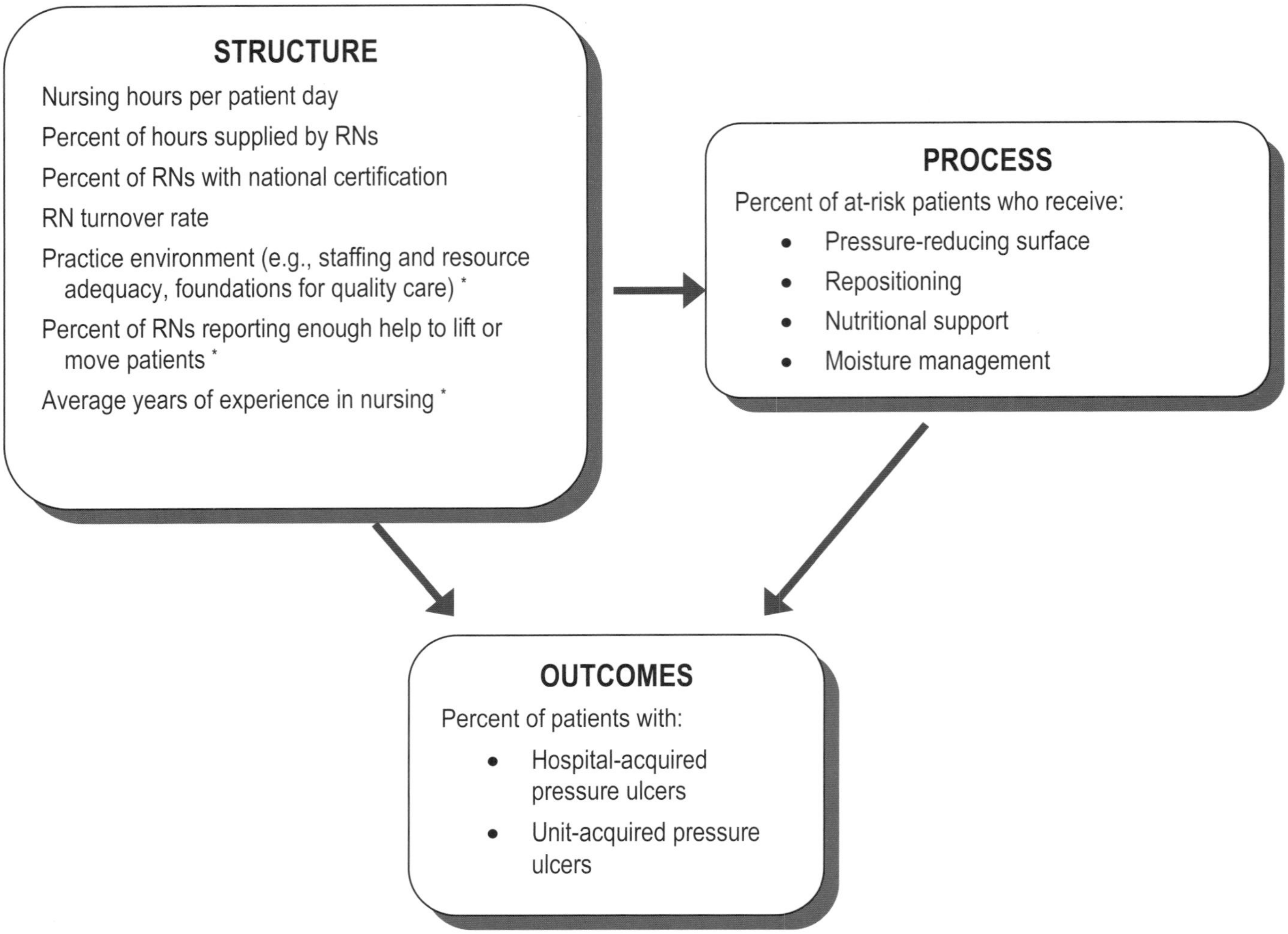

STRUCTURE

Nursing hours per patient day

Percent of hours supplied by RNs

Percent of RNs with national certification

RN turnover rate

Practice environment (e.g., staffing and resource adequacy, foundations for quality care) *

Percent of RNs reporting enough help to lift or move patients *

Average years of experience in nursing *

PROCESS

Percent of at-risk patients who receive:
- Pressure-reducing surface
- Repositioning
- Nutritional support
- Moisture management

OUTCOMES

Percent of patients with:
- Hospital-acquired pressure ulcers
- Unit-acquired pressure ulcers

Note: The direct relationship between structure and outcome is an NDNQI adaptation of Donabedian's (2003) linear proposition that structure influences process and process influences outcome.

★ Indicators from the annual RN Survey available to NDNQI-member hospitals.

have a falls problem even if they lack a protocol for evidence-based fall prevention. The same unit is likely to have many patients prone to developing pressure ulcers, requiring intensive prevention efforts to ensure good outcomes.

When using outcomes to evaluate nursing quality, stratification by unit type or statistical risk adjustment is a prerequisite to valid conclusions. A critical care unit's fall and pressure ulcer rates should be compared to other critical care units' rates, not to medical–surgical units' rates. Similarly, straight sums or averages of nursing units' outcomes to create hospital-wide measures of quality are fraught with inaccuracy and can obscure important differences in quality at the unit level. For example, if a hospital's three medical–surgical units had pressure ulcer rates of 0% but the hospital's critical care unit had a pressure ulcer rate of 14% (near the 75th

NDNQI Case Studies in Nursing Quality Improvement

percentile for NDNQI hospitals), the average rate at the hospital would be 3.5%. This hospital-wide pressure ulcer rate appears low, but hides the critical care unit's need for improvement and the success of the medical–surgical units. Thus, NDNQI outcome measures are stratified by unit type. Unit-type comparison data provided in NDNQI reports enables accurate conclusions about achievements or deficiencies in nursing care compared with peers.

Nurses engaged in quality improvement must make use of the relationship between structure, process, and outcomes. Structure and process indicators can help identify causes of poor outcomes, suggesting what corrective actions should be taken (Donabedian, 2003). Typically, changes in both the structure and process of care are required to optimize patient outcomes. For example, to reduce the percent of patients with hospital-acquired pressure ulcers (outcome), nurses will need to use evidence-based skin care protocols (process). But first they will need sufficient staffing levels and equipment (structure) to provide top-quality skin care. The structure of care is particularly important since it sets the stage for positive outcomes. NDNQI researchers have found that multiple aspects of nurse staffing (e.g., hours of nursing care, percent of RNs, and years of experience) are significantly related to patient falls and hospital-acquired pressure ulcers (Dunton, Gajewski, Klaus, & Pierson, 2007; Dunton, Gajewski, Taunton, & Moore, 2004). The way nursing care is structured affects what nurses do, which in turn affects patients' health.

Quality Improvement and Organizational Change

Most approaches to quality improvement (QI) share some core features. QI involves identifying problems, analyzing causes, testing solutions, evaluating progress, and making adjustments as needed. In many ways, QI is similar to the scientific method: hypotheses about the causes of deviation from ideal care are proposed, then tested with data to arrive at solutions to the original problem (Berwick, Godfrey, & Roessner, 1990; Donabedian, 2003).

Plan-Do-Check-Act (PDCA) is the most widely accepted method of improving quality. W. Edwards Deming popularized the method in the 1980s working with Japanese companies to increase productivity and market share (Deming, 1986). Today, PDCA is a useful guide for healthcare QI teams, and provides direction throughout a project.

In the first phase, nurses engaged in QI recognize an opportunity to improve and decide how to accomplish a change (Plan). Next, they carry out a test of the change on a small scale (Do). The effects of the change are observed (Check). Then the lessons learned from the test are used to revise the improvement plan or implement the changes on a broader scale (Act). Instead of "Check", some refer to the third phase as "Study", in order to accentuate the learning that should occur as a result of the test (Langley et al., 2009). The Institute for Healthcare Improvement (IHI) provides a Plan-Do-Study-Act worksheet to help quality improvement teams organize and learn from their efforts (IHI, 2010).

Langley et al. (2009) suggested three questions that should be asked, especially during the planning phase:

- What do we want to accomplish?

- How will we know if a change is actually an improvement?

- What changes can we make that will lead to improvement?

In the remaining phases of PDCA, changes tested in the real world provide nurses with knowledge they can use to improve quality on a larger, sustainable scale. Several rapid-cycle tests based on a "good enough" understanding of the problem may be useful in some situations. At other times, a more complete understanding and consensus among all parties may be needed before testing a change (Berwick, Godfrey, & Roessner, 1990). PDCA is useful for small- and large-scale unit-specific or hospital-wide initiatives.

PDCA proceeds in a circle or spiral. The PDCA cycle should be executed repeatedly for continued improvement (American Society for Quality, 2010). Each cycle leads to more knowledge and advanced quality of care, with each PDCA feeding into a new PDCA (see Figure 2). The continuous upward spiral of quality improvement results in superior patient, nurse, and hospital outcomes.

Other models of quality improvement are similar to PDCA but emphasize the broader context in which quality improvement occurs. For example, the United States Agency for International Development (USAID) uses the method shown in Figure 3 to improve healthcare services in developing countries (USAID, 2005). In this model, gaps between desired and actual performance are identified, interventions are selected to address the root causes of the gaps, and performance is continuously monitored to determine if the gaps are closing. All of this occurs within the organization's broader context, with stakeholder involvement maintained throughout.

Organizational context is the foundation on which QI rests. A hospital's culture especially affects nurses' ability to accomplish positive change. A culture of empowerment and accountability (responsibility, not blame), along with the pervasive belief that quality care ultimately reduces a hospital's costs, promotes continuous, effective QI. Successful improvement requires an openness to change and intentional, persistent efforts at all levels of the organization. Although unanimous agreement is unnecessary, stakeholder buy-in is required, from the direct-care nurses who will alter their practice, to the managers involved in planning and monitoring change, to the executives responsible for accomplishing the hospital's clinical and financial goals.

More than just a new checklist or a new policy is needed to improve the quality of nursing care. Staff need to be equipped and motivated for ongoing change. This book promotes continuous nursing quality improvement by equipping nurses with a "step-by-step" guide and real-life examples from 11 hospitals. Chapter 2 breaks down the steps contained within quality improvement methods.

References

All URLs retrieved December 10, 2010.

American Society for Quality. (2010). *Project planning and implementing tools: Plan-Do-Check-Act cycle.* http://www .asq.org/learn-about-quality/project-planning-tools/ overview/pdsa-cycle.html

Berwick, D. M., Godfrey, A. B., & Roessner, J. (1990). *Curing health care: New strategies for quality improvement.* San Francisco, CA: Jossey-Bass.

Centers for Medicare and Medicaid Services (CMS). (2010). *Reporting hospital quality data for annual payment update.* https://www.cms.gov/HospitalQualityInits/08_Hospital RHQDAPU.asp

Deming, W. E. (1986). *Out of the crisis.* Cambridge, MA: MIT Press.

Donabedian, A. (1966). Evaluating the quality of medical care. *The Milbank Memorial Fund Quarterly, 44*(3 Suppl.), 166–203.

Donabedian, A. (2003). *An introduction to quality assurance in health care.* New York, NY: Oxford University Press.

Dunton, N., Gajewski, B., Klaus, S., & Pierson, B. (2007). The relationship of nursing workforce characteristics to patient outcomes. *Online Journal of Issues in Nursing, 12*(3). http://www.nursingworld.org/MainMenuCategories/ ANAMarketplace/ANAPeriodicals/OJIN/Tableof Contents/Volume122007/No3Sept07/Nursing WorkforceCharacteristics.aspx

Dunton, N., Gajewski, B., Taunton, R. L., & Moore, J. (2004). Nurse staffing and patient falls on acute care hospital units. *Nursing Outlook, 52,* 53–59.

Institute for Healthcare Improvement (IHI). (2010). *Plan-Do-Study-Act (PDSA) worksheet.* http://www.ihi.org/ IHI/Topics/Improvement/ImprovementMethods/ Tools/Plan-Do-Study-Act%20(PDSA)%20Worksheet

Institute of Medicine (IOM). (2000). *To err is human: Building a safer health system.* Washington, DC: National Academies Press. http://www.iom.edu/Reports/1999/To-Err-is-Human-Building-A-Safer-Health-System.aspx

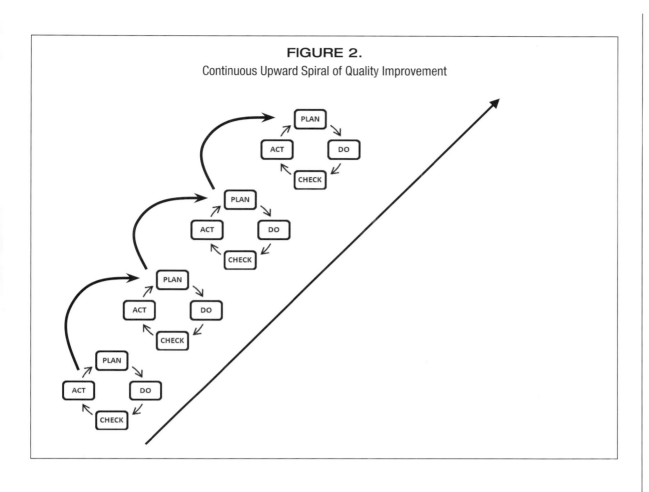

FIGURE 2.

Continuous Upward Spiral of Quality Improvement

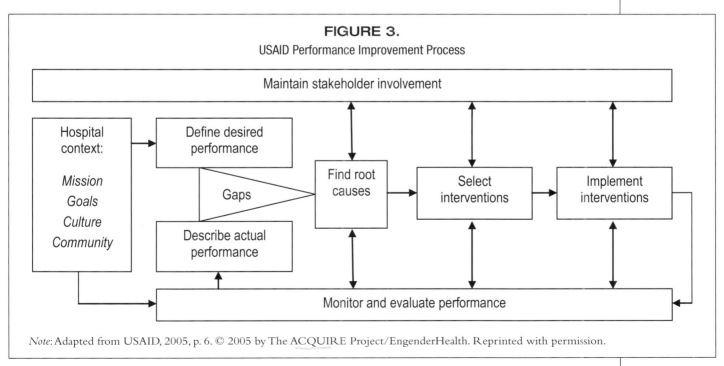

FIGURE 3.

USAID Performance Improvement Process

Maintain stakeholder involvement

Hospital context:

Mission
Goals
Culture
Community

Define desired performance

Gaps

Describe actual performance

Find root causes

Select interventions

Implement interventions

Monitor and evaluate performance

Note: Adapted from USAID, 2005, p. 6. © 2005 by The ACQUIRE Project/EngenderHealth. Reprinted with permission.

Institute of Medicine (IOM). (2001). *Crossing the quality chasm: A new health system for the 21st century*. Washington, DC: National Academies Press. http://www.iom.edu/Reports/2001/Crossing-the-Quality-Chasm-A-New-Health-System-for-the-21st-Century.aspx

Langley, G. J., Moen, R. D., Nolan, K. M., Nolan, T. W., Norman, C. L., & Provost, L. P. (2009). *The improvement guide* (2nd ed.). San Francisco, CA: Jossey-Bass.

Montalvo, I. (2007). The National Database of Nursing Quality Indicators (NDNQI). *Online Journal of Issues in Nursing, 12*(3). http://www.nursingworld.org/MainMenuCategories/ANAMarketplace/ANAPeriodicals/OJIN/TableofContents/Volume122007/No3Sept07/NursingQualityIndicators.aspx

Montalvo, I., & Dunton, N. (2007). *Transforming nursing data into quality care: Profiles of quality improvement in U.S. health-care facilities*. Silver Spring, MD: Nursesbooks.org.

National Quality Forum (NQF). (2004). *Nursing-sensitive care: Initial measures*. http://www.qualityforum.org/Projects/n-r/Nursing-Sensitive_Care_Initial_Measures/Nursing_Sensitive_Care_Initial_Measures.aspx

National Quality Forum (NQF). (2009). *Nursing-sensitive care: Measure maintenance*. http://www.qualityforum.org/Projects/n-r/Nursing-Sensitive_Care_Measure_Maintenance/Nursing_Sensitive_Care_Measure_Maintenance.aspx#t=1&s=&p=

United States Agency for International Development (USAID). (2005). *Guidance for program staff: Integrating best practices for performance improvement, quality improvement, and participatory learning and action to improve health services*. http://www.acquireproject.org/fileadmin/user_upload/ACQUIRE/Guidelines_pi_qi_pla_06-16-05.pdf

Chapter 2.
Using NDNQI Reports
for Quality Improvement

Effective quality improvement (QI) involves a series of steps or phases. Once a problem is identified, the QI team examines potential causes, then selects evidence-based structure and process remedies. Structure and process changes are implemented and adjusted as needed. Data from NDNQI® reports let nurses identify problem areas, explore possible causes, and monitor the effects of an improvement initiative. This chapter describes the QI steps (listed in Figure 1) and the role of NDNQI reports. Excerpts from the case studies in Chapter 3 are used to illustrate each step.

Over the years and across professions, authors have used various terms to describe the activities involved in quality improvement. Exact words and illustrations may vary, but all approaches to quality improvement share the same core elements. The particular author and the specific steps followed are less important than the use of an organized approach. An organized approach keeps the QI team focused and thorough, and helps to avoid reactionary changes made in an effort to quickly "do something". The steps described here fit within the PDCA cycle. The steps are "linear" (that is, they proceed in order), but the first and last steps are not the beginning and end. In practice, QI is ongoing and best thought of as an upward spiral.

Identify Problematic Areas

Opportunities for improvement can be identified in numerous ways: bedside staff input, audits of medical records, occurrence of a serious adverse event, deviations from usual performance, and comparison to peers. Consistent measurement of quality indicators is an efficient way to recognize gaps between actual and ideal performance. Data is the driving force behind problem identification.

The Restraint and Fall Committee examined monthly fall data and used NDNQI benchmarks to evaluate total and injury fall rates . . . The previous fall program was noted by staff and nursing leadership to no longer be effective. Multiple acute care nursing units had injury fall rates above the NDNQI mean in 3Q07 and there had been several falls with major injuries. (Memorial Hospital)

Visual tools that display repeated measures of an outcome over time (e.g., control charts) facilitate recognition of problematic areas (Langley et al., 2009). NDNQI graphs allow nurses to track their quality indicators over time, with the added benefit of comparison to peers. NDNQI comparison data features

---

FIGURE 1.
Steps Toward Improved Nursing Quality

- Identify problematic areas.
- Set measurable goals.
- Drill down to understand the problem.
- Examine structural factors.
- Identify successful nursing practices.
- Design the improvement plan.
- Implement the improvement plan.
  - Communicate.
  - Roll out.
  - Assess progress.
  - Adjust the plan.
  - Assess progress.
- Celebrate success!

percentiles, which are calculated from a rank ordering of units. For example, NDNQI analysts list the catheter-associated urinary tract infection (CAUTI) rates on adult critical care units in non-teaching hospitals from lowest to highest. The 75th percentile is the level at which 75% of these critical care units have lower CAUTI rates. In Figure 2, the 75th percentile is represented by the top of the gray bar. The critical care unit in this example often has CAUTI rates above the 75th percentile, which indicates a definite need for improvement.

NDNQI percentiles provide normative standards for judging quality. The nurse manager of a unit with injury falls rates consistently above the 50th percentile (the median) knows that over half of the unit's peers have fewer injury falls. Until 2008, NDNQI reports provided the mean instead of the median (50th per-

centile) for most indicators. Many hospitals used the mean (average) to identify problems. However, the mean is inflated when a few units have unusually high rates of adverse events. In such situations, the median is a more accurate reflection of "average" performance (Polit & Hungler, 1999). Therefore, *the median is preferred over the mean when evaluating patient outcomes*.

The NDNQI median represents "middle-of-the-road" quality. The 10th, 25th, 75th, and 90th percentiles in NDNQI reports provide the distribution of performance and can help identify the degree of a problem. A unit with hospital-acquired pressure ulcers (HAPUs) above the 75th percentile should recognize that 75% of their peers have better HAPU rates. Similarly, a pediatric unit whose average number of pain assessments is at the 10th percentile would understand that 90% of peer units provide more frequent pain assessments.

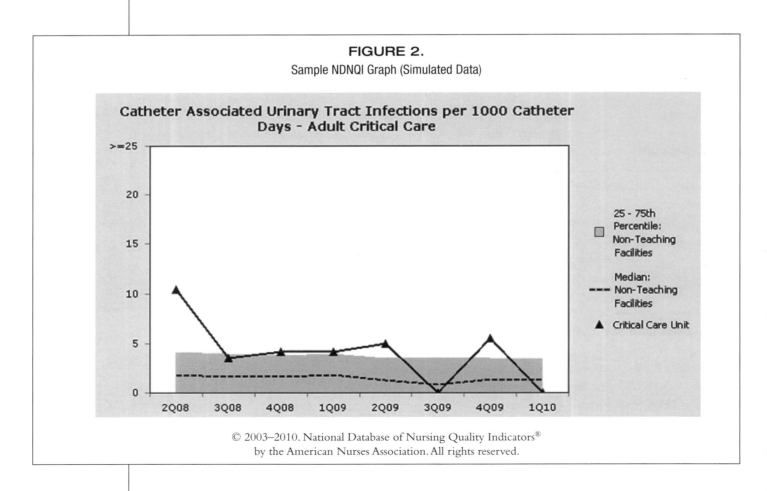

FIGURE 2.
Sample NDNQI Graph (Simulated Data)

Catheter Associated Urinary Tract Infections per 1000 Catheter Days - Adult Critical Care

**NDNQI Case Studies in
Nursing Quality Improvement**

Such reports should definitely spur these units to pursue the remaining QI steps described in this chapter.

HAPU rates in the intensive care units . . . were near the 90th percentile for NDNQI . . . in 2005 and 2006 . . . Subsequently, a series of changes in daily practice were used to promote a culture of HAPU prevention. (Scripps Memorial Hospital, La Jolla)

Once a problem is identified, a "process owner", someone who will be responsible for the entire improvement effort, should be selected. While support from hospital executives is necessary, the owner may be a manager or clinician who can lead the improvement (Berwick, Godfrey, & Roessner, 1990). The owner works with an interprofessional team to further define the problem, implement improvements, and measure progress. The team can be newly formed or an existing group (e.g., quality council) and can be unit-based or hospital-wide depending on the scope of the problem. Representatives from multiple professions (nursing, medicine, pharmacy, physical therapy, hospital resource management, etc.) and from multiple levels of the organization (unit managers, bedside nurses, executives) bring unique views and solutions to the problem. Hospitals often form and empower interprofessional outcome-specific teams (such as a pressure ulcer prevention team) to continually design, test, and implement changes.

The Best Practice Council identifies quality problems and creates interprofessional teams to review and test evidence-based practices. These smaller teams identify promising interventions and test them in the current environment to ensure positive impact. The team then makes recommendations to the larger Best Practice Council, which then mandates the practice change throughout the organization. The Patient Falls Prevention Team . . . included nursing staff and management, physical therapy, radiology, clinical nurse specialists, and nursing research. (St. Luke's Episcopal Hospital)

Before making any changes, the team should clearly define their purpose and examine possible causes of the problem. Setting goals and "drilling down" to the root of the problem are the next steps.

Set Measurable Goals

Goals keep a team focused and provide a ruler for measuring progress. Useful goals are quantifiable and specify the indicator, units, and timeframe. For example:

- Achieve injury falls rates below the NDNQI 25th percentile for medical–surgical units in Magnet® hospitals by 3Q11.

- Reduce the percent of critical care patients with unit-acquired pressure ulcers by half within six months.

- By March, patients on the pediatric surgical-trauma unit will be assessed for second-quarter pain hours in accordance with unit policy.

NDNQI reports provide ready-made goals. Percentiles tell you what qualifies as average, above average, and excellent quality (see Table 1). An acceptable mid-way goal is to reduce negative outcome rates to below the median. At the median (the middle), 50% of similar units have higher rates and 50% have lower rates. If a unit's total falls per 1,000 patient days had been above the 75th percentile, achieving fall rates below the median would represent a considerable improvement. However, the median does not necessarily represent ideal care. NDNQI percentiles are based on actual practice, with some hospitals attaining the desired goals of zero—e.g., for fall rates—not because the value is above average and is above the 50th percentile. Being at the median shows your quality of nursing care is "typical" or "average" compared to your peers.

For negative outcomes, above average quality is seen in the 25th percentile. A unit with catheter-associated urinary tract infections at or below the 25th percentile is in the top 25% of peers. Excellent care, or best practice, is reflected in the 10th percentile. A unit with total falls at or below the 10th percentile is in the top 10% of peers. For positive structure or process indicators such as RN hours per patient day, percent of

TABLE 1.

Guidelines for Evaluating Nursing Quality Measures Based on NDNQI Percentiles

Measure Direction	10th	25th	50th	75th	90th
Negative Measure (Falls, pressure ulcers, infections, nurse turn-over, nursing hours supplied by agency staff, etc.)	Excellent	Above average (Good)	Average	Below average	Poor
Positive Measure (Nursing hours supplied by RNs, certification, pediatric pain assessments, risk assessments, etc.)	Poor	Below average	Average	Above average (Good)	Excellent

Note: If it is a negative-directed measure, you want the numbers to go down. If it is a positive-directed measure, you want the numbers to go up.

RNs with certification, or pediatric pain assessment, the 90th percentile shows best practice.

> *Targets to continue reducing the rate of hospital-acquired pressure ulcers were established annually as follows:*
>
> > *FY07 = NDNQI mean or better*
> > *FY08 = NDNQI mean or better*
> > *FY09 = NDNQI 50th percentile or better*
> > *FY10 = NDNQI 25th percentile or better*
> > (Washington Hospital Center)

Drill Down to a Better Understanding

To design effective improvements, an examination of the problem and its causes is needed. The team should invest some time drilling down to the problem's core. In some cases, a problem's causes and solutions may be quite obvious. In others, a little digging may reveal an unexpected process at work.

> *Nursing leadership . . . quickly identified several key issues contributing to HAPU prevalence. The hospital had very limited expert resources, specifically 1.5 FTEs for Certified Wound, Ostomy, and Continence Nurses (CWOCN) for 530 beds. There was also a lack of knowledge among all staff, lack of bedside expertise, lack of standardized protocols, ineffective utilization of Braden scores, equipment issues, and inadequate communication of timely HAPU preva-*

> *lence data at the unit level.* (Shands Hospital at University of Florida)

> *As the PDCA team investigated the 2007 CAUTI cases, they found . . . patients who developed a CAUTI were most often those who were assessed to be a high fall risk. The team hypothesized that some of the infections were related to prolonged use of the catheter to decrease the patient's movement to the bathroom and mitigate a potential for a fall.* (Medical Center of the Rockies)

Information from multiple sources paints a clearer picture of the problem. The team can examine medical records, review patient satisfaction surveys, and interview or observe direct-care providers.

> *The team recognized the necessity of conducting an institutional needs assessment as their first step in improving pain management . . . Results from the survey of more than 300 staff demonstrated need for improvement in several areas, including standardized assessment and documentation . . . Of the patients and parents who responded to the team's survey, 28% responded that a pain rating scale was not used to assess pain.* (Advocate Hope Children's Hospital)

Health care has borrowed numerous analysis tools from the manufacturing industry (Graban, 2009; Ursprung & Gray, 2010). Tools such as root cause analysis and process mapping can reveal the sources of poor outcomes. For example, in root cause analysis, teams diagram the details of a specific case, then repeatedly ask, "Why did this happen?" until the underlying causes are exposed (Ursprung & Gray, 2010). Several authors have provided excellent guides for conducting effective root cause analyses (Pham et al., 2010; Ursprung & Gray, 2010).

NDNQI reports also help teams drill down. By examining NDNQI structure and process indicators, teams can identify factors contributing to undesirable patient outcomes. If a unit's total hours of nursing care per patient day is below the 25th percentile, or their use of agency personnel is higher than 90% of their peers, improved staffing may be part of the solution.

> *Exploration of the causes for the high [HAPU] rates included structural and process issues . . . During the first quarter of 2006 . . . 2G had a high staff turnover. Four temporary travel nurses were contracted to support staffing. The use of agency nurses was 11% that quarter. In addition, 2G staffing included four newly hired permanent RNs in orientation and two newly graduated RN hires . . . Staffing turbulence may have contributed to high pressure ulcer prevalence coupled with inconsistent knowledge and application of evidence-based practice for pressure ulcer prevention.* (Washington Hospital Center)

For outcomes such as falls and pressure ulcers, nursing care process indicators may reveal more about the problem. Figure 3 illustrates how data from NDNQI reports can help teams drill down on risk assessment and prevention interventions. On this unit, 16% of patients were not assessed for fall risk. Although 95% of the patients at risk had a prevention protocol in place, the unit's high fall rate suggests the protocol may need to be improved. The team should explore:

• What is preventing risk assessments?

• Is the risk assessment tool effective?

• Does the prevention program work?

Examining the nature of a quality problem paves the way for an effective improvement plan. However, two points should be kept in mind during the drill down phase. First, the improvement team should avoid lingering in analysis. Spending too much time defining the problem and its causes can actually hinder the pace of improvement (Berwick, Godfrey, & Roessner, 1990). Teams must balance the benefits of thorough understanding with the costs of inaction. When the problem and needed changes are exceedingly obvious, several authors recommend moving quickly toward implementing change (Berwick, Godfrey, & Roessner, 1990; Bornstein, 2001). Second, teams need a strong bias toward a systems view of the problem (Crigger, 2005). Drill down focuses on the changes needed to correct faulty systems and promote consistently positive outcomes. Ideally, drill down occurs within a "just culture", in which problems are openly acknowledged, processes are redesigned to reduce the likelihood of error, and, when indicated, individuals are disciplined for reckless or malevolent behavior (Marx, 2001).

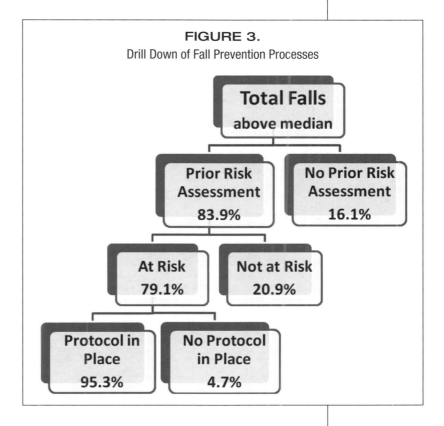

FIGURE 3.
Drill Down of Fall Prevention Processes

Focusing on faulty systems does not negate individual accountability for practice; rather, it makes people accountable for recognizing and correcting unsafe systems (Crigger, 2005; Marx, 2001).

As an understanding of the quality problem and its causes unfold, teams should begin their search for evidence-based remedies. Improvements to both the structure and processes of care should be explored in the next two steps.

Examine Structural Factors

Structural factors facilitate or hinder nurses' ability to provide quality care. Teams who find ways to improve the structure of care set the stage for better outcomes. Staffing, supplies, and organizational culture are essential structural factors that influence the processes of care and patient outcomes.

Numerous studies have shown higher RN hours per patient day are associated with better patient outcomes (Aiken, Clarke, Sloane, Sochalski, & Silber, 2002; Dall, Chen, Seifert, Maddox, & Hogan, 2009; Kane, Shamliyan, Mueller, Duval, & Wilt, 2007; Needleman, Bauerhaus, Mattke, Stewart, & Zelevinsky, 2002). Staffing mix (percent of nursing care hours supplied by RNs, unlicensed assistive personnel, and agency staff), education, and certification also affect the quality of nursing care a unit can provide (Blegen & Vaughn, 1998; Cho, Ketefian, Barkauskas, & Smith, 2003; Kane et al., 2007; Needleman et al., 2002). Beyond the number and type of nurses on a unit, staff expertise is a key structural factor. Placing experts at the bedside can be an effective strategy in combating negative outcomes.

In order to eliminate the use of travelers, administration made a commitment to hire Student Nurse Externs (SNEs) with the expectation that a majority of these students would remain after graduation . . . Additionally, managers in the medical-surgical areas were instructed to over-hire RNs by 20% with the understanding that they would be "feeder" units for the ICU intern training program . . . To assist staff

nurses with reducing pressure ulcers, an ICU Wound Care Nurse was hired two days per week. (Scripps Memorial Hospital, La Jolla)

When looking at potential causes of the infections it became clear that there was no consistency in how any of the central lines were managed. Over 50 physicians and neonatal nurse practitioners were able to place peripherally inserted central catheters (PICCs) . . . A proposal for a dedicated unit-based line insertion team consisting of two full-time nurses was presented. (Cook Children's Medical Center)

Nursing leadership embraced the Ostomy Wound Liaison (OWL) resource nurse model to empower frontline nursing staff to improve their practice and patient outcomes . . . In 2006, six Clinical Nurse Specialist (CNS) positions were implemented . . . The new CNSs mentored the unit-based OWL resource nurses . . . The OWLs conduct rounds and develop individualized plans of care . . . They are recognized as skin care experts by their peers and physician colleagues. (Shands Hospital at the University of Florida)

Teams should also identify the supplies needed to provide top quality care. New equipment such as bed alarms, pressure-reducing mattresses, or central-line dressing kits may need to be purchased. Especially as reimbursement for some reasonably preventable hospital-acquired conditions is no longer provided by the Centers for Medicare and Medicaid Services (CMS) and many private insurers, the cost savings of preventing injury falls, pressure ulcers, and device-associated infections typically outweighs the costs of new equipment or additional staff.

The Weekly Falls Review Team identified the need to enhance the sensitivity of existing bed alarms with the purchase of conversion kits . . . Since there are often more patients at high risk for falls than there are rooms in close proximity to the nurses' station, the team determined that 24 rooms throughout the various nursing units would benefit from surveillance cameras and grant money was used for their purchase.

Finally, in order to eliminate the cause of some falls during the use of bedside commodes, the team proposed the purchase of bedside commodes with drop sides to ease patient movement onto the equipment. (CHRISTUS St. Michael Health System)

The improved patient outcomes leading to an estimated savings of $7,590,000 were tied to the ongoing availability of personnel and material resources, namely retaining a dedicated CWOCN for adult critical care and approving the purchase of turning wedges and heel protectors. (St. John Medical Center)

An organization's culture can have powerful, if sometimes unnoticed, influences on nursing-sensitive outcomes. Anything from leadership effectiveness to prevailing philosophies of care to bedside nurses' involvement in decision making can be appropriate targets for structural change.

The intensive care units . . . were considered one unit, led by one manager who oversaw 41 beds and more than 120 employees. The manager's effectiveness was limited by a large span of control covering multiple, geographically separate units . . . The intensive care units were separated into three specialty units in the spring of 2007 and two additional managers were hired. This improved managerial effectiveness and increased staff expertise for a specific patient population. (Scripps Memorial Hospital, La Jolla)

The resource nurse model also served as an effective strategy for empowering all bedside staff. Bedside nurses understand clinical issues and will find practical and creative solutions. For example, because of the length of time CICU [Cardiac Intensive Care Unit] patients spend in the operating room and their instability post-operatively, the CICU staff noted that their patients needed to be placed on the correct bed surface immediately in the OR. They arranged to take the appropriate bed to the OR suite so the patient could be transferred from the operating table directly onto the bed. (Shands Hospital at the University of Florida)

By searching the literature, gathering examples of success from peers (at professional meetings such as the annual NDNQI conference, for instance), and drawing on the expertise of quality organizations (IHI, Agency for Healthcare Research and Quality, etc.), teams can find evidence-based ways to improve the structure of nursing care. These same sources of evidence apply when identifying successful nursing practices.

Identify Successful Nursing Practices

Nursing practices (processes of nursing care) comprise all the things nurses do as they provide care, such as assess patients, intervene to prevent and treat patient conditions, and educate patients and families. Coordinating care, documenting, and making rounds are also processes of nursing care that influence patient outcomes. To reach the goal a team has set, multiple processes will likely need improvement. Teams that not only select evidence-based preventive interventions but also focus on efficiency and reduction of non-patient care tasks will have the greatest impact on patient, nurse, and financial outcomes.

Evidence-based practice recommendations stated that removal of the urinary catheter as early as possible is very effective in CAUTI prevention . . . The PDCA team submitted their recommendation for daily review of catheter necessity with the goal of implementing culture changes that supported the best practice of removing urinary catheters within 3 days of insertion . . . In the new process, review of catheter necessity was to be facilitated by the patient's assigned RN in collaboration with the patient's physician during interprofessional team rounds each day. (Medical Center of the Rockies)

As of early 2007, charting pain management required access to three separate areas of the Patient Care Flowsheet as well as electronic charting on medication administration. Revisions to the daily nursing documentation form were made to co-locate all pain assessment data for a more logical flow of information. In addition, coded lists of common pain management interventions were provided, rather than having to repeatedly write out common interventions. (Children's Hospital of Philadelphia)

Selecting meaningful risk-assessment tools and then linking prevention interventions to a patient's risk can result in improved outcomes. Many negative outcomes are preventable if the right patients are given the right interventions (Clark, 2010). Teams can search for or develop easy-to-complete assessment tools and corresponding order sets or plans of care.

Staff stated the assessment tools were cumbersome and that "most patients became fall risks" based on the criteria used. After further discussion and analysis, it was concluded that most patients . . . are at risk for falls, which generated discussion of a two-tier fall prevention process. The first tier utilizes the concept of "standard" fall precautions for all acute care patients . . . At the second tier, patients would be placed on "strict" fall precautions. (Memorial Hospital)

The hospital's WOCN clinical specialist revised the skin assessment tool to include the Braden Score and a guide to various skin care products . . . This assessment tool streamlined skin care documentation onto one flowsheet and assisted nurses in selecting appropriate interventions. (Washington Hospital Center)

Evidence-based intervention bundles and clinical guidelines are available from numerous sources (see Appendix B). For example, the Improvement Map from the Institute for Healthcare Improvement lists five processes known to reduce central line-associated blood stream infections: hand hygiene, barrier precautions upon insertion, chlorohexadine antisepsis, optimal site selection, and daily review of line necessity (IHI, 2010). Teams can adopt these proven processes with confidence, saving the effort of selecting individual strategies from the original research literature.

Design the Improvement Plan

From the structural factors and successful nursing practices that have been identified, the team designs a focused, evidence-based improvement plan. Each plan will be unique to the hospital or unit and will directly target the causes of the problem that the team has identified. Adopting research-supported interventions along with innovative strategies successfully used by peers is likely to result in a cost-effective improvement plan that produces results.

The plan will include both structure and process changes, since both are determinants of patient outcomes. Hospitals and units featured in the case studies used multiple structure and process interventions to improve their nursing-sensitive outcomes. The improvement plan should also contain a general timeline and should outline strategies for implementing the changes in practice, including communicating with, motivating, and educating staff. Direct-care staff participation on the team designing the plan enhances feasibility and buy-in. Teams can also solicit feedback about the plan from staff who will be asked to change their practice, or gain approval from a shared governance council.

Implement the Improvement Plan

Implementation encompasses the "Do-Check-Act" phases of the PDCA cycle. Before any changes are made, the first thing to "Do" is communicate with and educate staff about the structure and processes that will be changing. Numerous techniques and venues can be used (posters, emails, newsletters, meetings or in-services, online training modules, etc.). Vision, motivation, and accountability will be especially critical to success.

The clinical educator and CWOCN developed timelines for implementation and a theme which was gender neutral and engaged all staff. The AICU's [Adult Intensive Care Unit's] War on Wounds was announced to staff: "YOU have been called to duty. MISSION—SAVE OUR PATIENTS' SKIN". The strategies became the "battle plan". This information was communicated during staff meetings and unit-based council meetings. Periodic progress reports were posted on the QI board for all to see. When the manual turning strategy was implemented, overhead announcements were made to remind staff to turn their patients. (St. John Medical Center)

SICU [Surgical Intensive Care Unit] staff nurses worked on designing posters to provide staff education related to "why" the change in practice was needed and "how" to measure the change. Training was focused on providing "world-class" patient care, with patient safety, comfort, and reduction of infection as the goal. Posters that explained the new procedure were displayed in places that would catch staff attention . . . SICU RNs who were members of the Standards of Care (SOC) Committee communicated the policy revisions and goals for CAUTI reduction to all nursing staff through emails, flyers, posters, and staff meetings. An incentive of a meal for staff (such as pizza for all shifts) was offered if the unit was able to decrease the incidence of CAUTI by 75% when the review of results occurred in July. (Medical Center of the Rockies)

The second thing to do is to roll out the plan. New staff may have been hired, documentation and supply systems revised, and new policies and procedures created. In the overlap between the design and implementation steps, the QI team arranges the details of each change. Subsequently, all these changes go into practice. Implementation can occur all at once or phase by phase, depending on the complexity of the changes being made. Pilot testing the changes on one or two units before implementing hospital-wide allows teams to adapt the plan as needed, saving resources and preventing unnecessary upheaval.

New risk-assessment tools and "traffic light" signs were trialed on two units with high-risk populations and increased fall rates . . . After the trial, nursing staff said that the new fall signage was helpful . . . However, they stated the assessment tools were cumbersome . . . After the Nurse Practice Council provided feedback regarding the two-tier program changes, the program was re-piloted . . . [then] rolled out via education through an electronic module . . . The program went live hospital-wide after education in March 2008. (Memorial Hospital)

Next, data returns to the forefront as teams "Check" how well the new structures and processes of care are working. By continuing to collect data according to NDNQI protocol, teams can determine if their plan has had the desired impact. Many units decide to monitor their progress monthly during an improvement initiative. Frequent data collection facilitates timely revisions to the improvement plan.

Along with the OWL resource nurse model, monthly prevalence studies have proved to be a breakthrough strategy for the Pressure Ulcer Prevention team . . . the methodical data collection process serves not only as a means to calculate HAPU rates, but also to identify problems that need to be addressed. (Shands Hospitals at the University of Florida)

Other things besides the improvement plan can affect outcome rates. Random fluctuations in patient severity, unit census, staff turnover, or other unanticipated changes on the unit that were not part of the plan can "accidentally" lower or increase outcome rates. To the extent possible, keep everything else on the unit the same during a pilot test. All quality indicators are subject to "regression to the mean," a statistical name for the idea that over time, things tend to even out. For example, a unit that has several months or quarters of high fall rates is quite likely to see their rates drop the next quarter, no matter what they do. For this reason, one or two data points do not prove or disprove a plan's effectiveness. Teams must continue to track data over several months and quarters to look for evidence of real improvement.

Graphing the data will help teams visualize actual shifts in performance. Graphs such as run charts and control charts are especially useful. Run charts allow teams to determine if changes have resulted in improvement (Langley et al., 2009). A run chart plots data points in chronological order, with the median of these data points as a reference line. As illustrated in Figure 4, the presence of six or more consecutive data points on the lower side of the unit's median provides solid evidence that changes in nursing structure and processes have improved patient outcomes (Langley et al., 2009). When evaluating the effects of a quality improvement

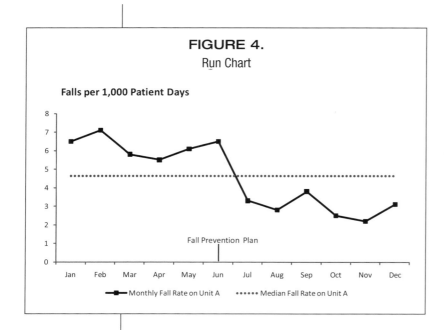

FIGURE 4.
Run Chart

Falls per 1,000 Patient Days

Fall Prevention Plan

■— Monthly Fall Rate on Unit A　••••• Median Fall Rate on Unit A

plan, the run chart is preferable to other tools such as bar graphs or superimposed trend lines, since run charts show when a meaningful change has occurred (Balestracci, 2009, 2010).

Control charts facilitate the evaluation of how stable a process is and identify common cause or special cause variation (Harris, 1999; Langley et al., 2009). Common cause variation refers to random differences between

data points. Special cause variation occurs when a specific change (such as the improvement plan) produces a meaningful difference between data points. A control chart plots data in chronological order, adding a center line plus upper and lower control limits. In Figure 5, wide fluctuations in HAPU during 2007 and 2008 are due to common cause variation; the same nursing processes produced these data points. The improved pressure ulcer rates beginning in 2009 are due to a special cause. Formulas for calculating control limits depend on the type of data collected (Langley et al., 2009). Many other resources are available to further explore the use of control charts for quality improvement purposes.

Additional improvements beyond the original plan are often needed to reach previously set goals. If graphs reveal that pressure ulcer, infection, or fall rates are unchanged or at least not improved to the degree desired, teams repeat the earlier steps: hypothesize why outcomes remain elevated, select appropriate structure and processes changes, roll out the additional interventions, and assess progress. No plan is carved in stone; interventions may be revised or added. Flexibility and persistence are keys to success.

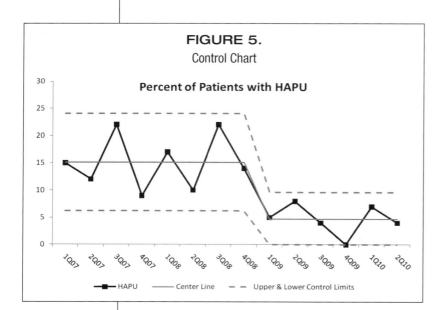

FIGURE 5.
Control Chart

Percent of Patients with HAPU

■— HAPU　—— Center Line　– – Upper & Lower Control Limits

By October 2008 there did not seem to be an appreciable decrease in patient falls despite the implementation of the evidence-based Falls Prevention Protocol. The existing Falls Committee . . . met to brainstorm what else could be done. Another committee had successfully reduced length of stay by instituting weekly review of every case in which patients were hospitalized longer than five days. The Falls Committee asked themselves, "Why can't we meet every week as well, to review every patient fall?" Thus, CHRISTUS St. Michael established an interprofessional Weekly Falls Review Team . . . to identify preventable causes of falls . . . A downward trend in the raw number of monthly falls began immediately following creation of the Weekly Falls Review Team. (CHRISTUS St. Michael Health System)

Despite the changes initiated prior to 2007, the annual HAPU rate only decreased from 21.6% to

NDNQI Case Studies in
Nursing Quality Improvement

19.7%, still above the NDNQI mean for comparable hospitals . . . Analysis of prevalence data and root causes led to a series of systematic rapid improvement cycles using the Plan-Do-Check-Act (PDCA) model concentrating on culture, workforce, products, and education . . . the unit experienced progressively more quarters with fewer than 10% Stage II HAPU. By 2009, the SICU's annual rate declined to 6.6%. (Scripps Memorial Hospital, La Jolla)

Celebrate Success

When improvement is achieved, celebrate! Acknowledging small and large gains instills pride in quality care and creates a positive culture. Celebrating success also helps sustain improvement and motivate future initiatives. This is by no means the final step. In the ever-changing world of daily patient care, quality improvement is continuous. But celebrating milestones is an important step in the ongoing cycle.

The NICU [Neonatal Intensive Care Unit] has been able to make CLABSI [central line-associated blood stream infection] prevention part of the unit culture rather than just another QI project. Since combating CLABSIs is a never-ending process, the unit will continue to strive for the only acceptable rate: zero. The current number of infection-free days is electronically displayed for staff members to see as they enter each lounge. When the unit reached 100 days infection-free, each staff member received a candy bar with a homemade wrapper that states "Hooray 100 days infection free". When the unit reached 200 days, the hospital patient safety officer supplied the staff with a pizza party to celebrate that success. The NICU has had so much success that other units in the hospital as well as other neonatal ICUs around the area have requested information on the NICU's practices . . . The PICC team has traveled to evaluate other hospitals and give feedback on their current practice and suggestions for how to improve. NICU leaders and staff will keep working to maintain the success, share the story, and learn from others as the journey continues. (Cook Children's Medical Center)

References

All URLs retrieved December 10, 2010.

Aiken, L. H., Clarke, S. P., Sloane, D. M., Sochalski, J., & Silber, J. H. (2002). Hospital nurse staffing and patient mortality, nurse burnout, and job dissatisfaction. *Journal of the American Medical Association, 288,* 1987–1993.

Balestracci, D. (2009). *Data sanity: A quantum leap to unprecedented results.* Englewood, CO: Medical Group Management Association.

Balestracci, D. (2010). *Data sanity: Introduction to good, basic measurement skills.* ANA Webinar. http://eo2.commpartners.com/users/aname/archived.php

Berwick, D. M., Godfrey, A. B., & Roessner, J. (1990). *Curing health care: New strategies for quality improvement.* San Francisco, CA: Jossey-Bass.

Blegen, M. A., & Vaughn, T. (1998). A multisite study of nurse staffing and patient occurrences. *Nursing Economic$, 16*(4), 196–203.

Bornstein, T. (2001). *Quality improvement and performance improvement: Different means to the same end?* http://www.reproline.jhu.edu/english/6read/6pi/pi_qi/piqi1.htm

Cho, S., Ketefian, S., Barkauskas, V. H., & Smith, D. G. (2003). The effects of nurse staffing on adverse events, morbidity, mortality, and medical costs. *Nursing Research, 52*(2), 71–79.

Clark, C. (2010). Simple "three bucket" tool helps prevent huge cause of inpatient death. *HealthLeaders Media.* http://www.healthleadersmedia.com/content/COM-252215/Simple-Three-Bucket-Tool-Helps-Prevent-Huge-Cause-of-Inpatient-Death

Crigger, N. (2005). Two models of mistake-making in professional practice: Moving out of the closet. *Nursing Philosophy, 6,* 11–18.

Dall, T. M., Chen, Y. J., Seifert, R. F., Maddox, P. J., & Hogan, P. F. (2009). The economic value of professional nursing. *Medical Care, 47*(1), 97–104.

Graban, M. (2009). *Lean hospitals: Improving quality, patient safety, and employee satisfaction.* Boca Raton, FL: CRC Press.

Harris, R. L. (1999). *Information graphics: A comprehensive illustrated reference.* New York, NY: Oxford University Press.

Institute for Healthcare Improvement (IHI). (2010). *IHI improvement map: Central line bundle.* http://www.ihi.org/imap/tool/#Process=e876565d-fd43-42ce-8340-8643b7e675c7

Kane, R. L., Shamliyan, T., Mueller, C., Duval, S., & Wilt, T. J. (2007). *Nurse staffing and quality of patient care.* U.S. Department of Health and Human Services. http://www.ahrq.gov/downloads/pub/evidence/pdf/nurse-staff/nursestaff.pdf

Langley, G. J., Moen, R. D., Nolan, K. M., Nolan, T. W., Norman, C. L., & Provost, L. P. (2009). *The improvement guide: A practical approach to enhancing organizational performance* (2nd ed.). San Francisco, CA: Jossey-Bass.

Marx, D. (2001). *Patient safety and the "just culture": A primer for healthcare executives.* (April 17. Prepared by David Marx, JD, for Columbia University under a grant provided by the National Heart, Lung, and Blood Institute.) Trustees of Columbia University: New York, NY. http://www.mers-tm.org/support/Marx_Primer.pdf

Needleman, J., Buerhaus, P., Mattke, S., Steward, M., & Zelevinsky, K. (2002). Nurse-staffing levels and the quality of care in hospitals. *New England Journal of Medicine, 346,* 1715–1722.

Pham, J. C., Kim, G. R., Natterman, J. P., Cover, R. M., Goeschel, C. A., Wu, A. W., & Provonost, P. J. (2010). ReCASTing the RCA: An improvement model for performing root cause analyses. *American Journal of Medical Quality, 25*(3), 186–191.

Polit, D. F., & Hungler, B. P. (1999). *Nursing research: Principles and methods* (6th ed.). Philadelphia, PA: Lippincott Williams & Wilkins.

Ursprung, R., & Gray, J. (2010). Random safety auditing, root cause analysis, failure mode and effects analysis. *Clinics in Perinatology, 37,* 141–165.

Chapter 3.
Case Studies in
Quality Improvement

NDNQI® invited 11 hospitals to share their stories of successful nursing quality improvement in this chapter. Hospitals were selected by two methods. First, regression analysis was used to rank all NDNQI nursing units based on the degree of improvement in their indicators from the second quarter of 2007 to the first quarter of 2009. The units in the top 10% that maintained improvement for at least three quarters were grouped by hospital to identify potential candidates for case studies. Second, several hospitals that presented posters at the 2009 NDNQI conference about structure and process changes that led to improved outcomes were asked to retell their stories here.

The case studies cover improvements in pressure ulcers, patient falls, hospital-acquired infections, and pediatric pain assessment. A wide variety of hospital and unit types are represented. The case studies demonstrate the quality improvement steps discussed in Chapter 2, telling:

- How problems were identified;

- How structure and process interventions were selected and implemented;

- How progress was monitored; and

- How improvements were achieved, sustained, and celebrated.

Through these case studies, we hope nurses will gain ideas and inspiration for improving care on their units.

Pressure Ulcers

Utilizing a Resource Nurse Model to Improve Nosocomial Pressure Ulcer Rates

War on Wounds in the Adult Intensive Care Units

Comprehensive Pressure Ulcer Prevention Program Improves Outcomes for At-Risk Patients

Incremental Changes in Culture, Workforce, and Products Reduce Hospital-Acquired Pressure Ulcers in the Intensive Care Setting

Patient Falls

Weekly Falls Review Team: Nurse-Driven Interprofessional Initiative to Decrease Patient Falls in the Acute Care Setting

Two-Tier Fall Precautions Combined with Improved Staffing and New Equipment Reduce Injury Fall Rates

Multiple Practice Changes Promote a Culture of Shared Responsibility to Reduce Patient Falls and Fall Injuries

Hospital-Acquired Infections

Reducing Catheter-Associated Urinary Tract Infections in the Surgical Intensive Care Unit

Primary Line Insertion Team Reduced Central Line-Associated Blood Stream Infections in the Neonatal ICU

Pediatric Pain Assessment

Pain Resource Nurse Program and Monthly Chart Audits Improve Pediatric Pain Assessment

Improving Pain Assessment and Management on Pediatric Medical–Surgical Units

Utilizing a Resource Nurse Model to Improve Nosocomial Pressure Ulcer Rates

Gale Danek, PhD, RN, NE-BC
Administrative Director, Nursing Research
danekg@shands.ufl.edu

Betty Jax, MSN, ARNP, RN-BC
Administrative Director, Nursing Education

Peggy Guin, PhD, ARNP, CNRN, CNS-BC
Neuroscience Clinical Nurse Specialist

Shands Hospital at the University of Florida
Gainesville, Florida
www.shands.org/hospitals/uf/

Case Study Highlights

Unit staff nurses were trained as Ostomy Wound Liaison (OWL) resource nurses to serve as pressure ulcer prevention experts for their peers. OWLs collaborated with the hospital's Pressure Ulcer Prevention (PUP) Team to implement product and process changes. Monthly prevalence studies facilitated immediate remedy of pressure ulcer causes. These strategies, characterized by team building and staff empowerment, led to sustained improvement in hospital-acquired pressure ulcer (HAPU) rates.

Pressure Ulcers in Highly Complex Patients

In early 2004, the Nursing Quality Council and nursing leadership at Shands Hospital at the University of Florida (SUF) recognized that the hospital lacked a reliable measure for assessing pressure ulcer issues.

Although SUF has participated in NDNQI® since 2002 (see Figure 1), pressure ulcer data were not submitted until 2004. At this time, SUF committed to conducting quarterly pressure ulcer prevalence studies and submitting data to NDNQI. One of the driving forces for doing this was the confidence that NDNQI comparison data would provide accurate benchmarks for the hospital's complex and high-acuity patient populations.

In 2004, adult intensive care and intermediate care patients made up 30% of the total beds and were the highest risk patients for pressure ulcer development. In the first quarter of 2004 (1Q04), SUF's four adult intensive care units (ICUs) had an average HAPU prevalence of 23.8%, well above the NDNQI mean of 17.5% for ICUs in hospitals with over 500 beds.

The cardiac intensive care unit (CICU), which cares for cardiac and cardiothoracic surgical patients (see Figure 2), had a much higher HAPU rate at 37.5%.

FIGURE 1.
Facility Profile

Shands Hospital at the University of Florida (SUF)
Gainesville, Florida
www.shands.org/hospitals/uf/

Facility overview	Shands Hospital at the University of Florida is the flagship hospital for Shands HealthCare, a private healthcare system with seven hospitals, two home health agencies, and 80 affiliated outpatient practices. In November 2009, SUF opened a new Cancer and Critical Care Hospital on the south campus, which increased SUF's licensed beds from 660 to 852. Approximately 1,500 UF faculty and community physicians provide care in 100 specialty and subspecialty medical areas, including centers of excellence for cancer, cardiovascular, neurology, neurosurgery, pediatrics, and transplantation services. SUF has participated in NDNQI since 2002.
Teaching status	Academic medical center
Ownership status	Not-for-profit
Magnet® status	Magnet-designated since 2003
Staffed beds	819
Affiliations	University of Florida Shands HealthCare
Awards	Florida Governor's Sterling Award (Shands Healthcare), 2008 American Stroke Association's Gold Award, 2010 Increasing the Capacity to Care Nursing Award (Rubbermaid Medical Solutions), 2010

FIGURE 2.
Unit Profile

Overview The Cardiac Intensive Care Unit (CICU) is divided into four six-bed "pods". One pod houses clinically unstable cardiac medicine patients; the other three house cardiothoracic surgery patients with complex heart surgeries or status-post heart transplant. CICU received the AACN Beacon Award for Excellence in 2009.

Unit	Staffed Beds	Total NHPPD[a]	Hours Supplied by RNs (%)	RNs with BSN Degree (%)	RNs with National Certification (%)	Average RN Experience (years)
CICU	24	18.3	100	51	1.2[b]	8.3

Notes:

[a] NHPPD = Nursing hours per patient day.

[b] Certification was 1.2% when the HAPU problem was identified; the unit's NDNQI report for 4Q09 shows certification is now 27.9%.

NDNQI Case Studies in Nursing Quality Improvement

Many CICU patients have overall poor perfusion and are particularly prone to pressure damage. Cardiovascular surgery patients posed the highest risk. These patients had operating room times that frequently exceeded eight hours and many required extended use of cardiac bypass or aortic cross-clamp during surgery. CICU patients with dissecting aortic aneurysms virtually lost perfusion below the point of the dissection until surgical repair could be completed. Routine HAPU prevention strategies were more difficult to execute in CICU patients because of the presence of multiple IV/IA access devices or open chest cavities. As a result, the culture on the CICU prior to 2004 was somewhat resigned, as the staff viewed HAPUs as an unavoidable complication of that population.

Initial Response to High HAPU Rates

The initial HAPU reduction activities in 2004 and 2005 centered on understanding the issues and helping staff "own" the problem. Nursing leadership, particularly the Vice President of Nursing and the Administrative Director for Professional Practice, quickly identified several key issues contributing to HAPU prevalence. The hospital had very limited expert resources, specifically 1.5 full-time employees (FTEs) for Certified Wound, Ostomy, and Continence Nurses (CWOCN) for 530 beds. There was also a lack of knowledge among all staff, lack of bedside expertise, lack of standardized protocols, ineffective utilization of Braden scores, equipment issues, and inadequate communication of timely HAPU prevalence data at the unit level.

NDNQI quarterly prevalence studies helped address several issues. The data collection process was standardized, staff became more aware of HAPUs, and valid benchmarking data allowed nursing leadership to set goals for the hospital and each unit. HAPUs became the first nursing-sensitive indicator fully embraced by unit level staff, nursing leadership, and senior administration. In late 2004, Shands Healthcare launched a system-wide Pressure Ulcer Prevention (PUP) Team initiative that served to solidify top administrative support and goal setting. Evidence-based skin care protocols were developed and extensive staff education was implemented. SUF's PUP team was led by an administrative director and the CWOCN. By 4Q05, the average HAPU prevalence rates on the adult ICUs improved to 6.4%, with CICU dramatically reducing their rate to 4.7%.

The Resource Nurse Model

Although significant progress was made over the initial two years, nursing leadership realized in early 2006 that further efforts were required to consistently hold the gains from quarter to quarter. If staff were to own this nursing-sensitive indicator, a creative strategy was needed. Consistent with Magnet® philosophy and the SUF nursing vision of "autonomous, accountable nursing practice", senior nursing leadership embraced the Ostomy Wound Liaison (OWL) resource nurse model to empower frontline nursing staff to improve their practice and patient outcomes.

The OWL resource nurse model had initially been piloted on a few ICUs in 2004. In 2006, six clinical nurse specialist (CNS) positions were implemented. The CNSs were involved in expanding the OWL program to all units, including critical care, medical-surgical, and pediatric areas. Along with the CWOCN, the new CNSs mentored the unit-based resource nurses.

Resource nurses, as defined by SUF leadership, are clinical experts who function as both a resource and a change agent by disseminating evidence-based information and interfacing with nurses, physicians, patients, and families. For staff nurses to become resources and change agents for their peers, they must receive advanced education, develop their clinical and interpersonal skills, and spend time practicing with clinical experts. To accomplish this, several strategies were established:

- Basic OWL training consisting of a one-day education session with CWOCNs and experienced

OWLs and completion of NDNQI pressure ulcer online training

- Rounds with experienced OWLs, CWOCNs, or CNSs

- Participation in monthly prevalence studies, with CWOCNs or CNSs verifying all ulcers and ulcer staging to increase confidence in data accuracy

- Clinical practicum with CWOCNs or experienced OWLs

- One-day courses focusing on interpersonal skills and change strategies

- Quarterly education meetings

- Yearly Wound and Skin Continuing Education Days

- Ongoing mentoring by CWOCNs and CNSs to help resource nurses synthesize information and operationalize their role at the bedside

Upon completion of the basic OWL training, new resource nurses receive the OWL recognition pin (see Figure 3). Designed jointly by the CWOCNs and OWLs, the pin enables colleagues to easily identify the resource nurses.

FIGURE 3.
OWL Recognition Pin

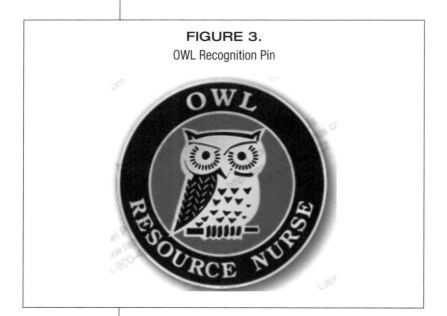

Keys to Success: Teamwork and Empowerment

Throughout implementation of the OWL program, the interprofessional PUP team established in 2004 continued to lead pressure ulcer prevention. Along with an OWL representative from each unit, PUP team members include a physician, a physical therapist, and a dietitian. In 2008, two staff nurse OWLs became co-chairs of the team, with a CWOCN and a CNS serving as advisers. The PUP team has been engaged in ongoing quality improvement, including:

- Review of monthly prevalence data with comparison to NDNQI benchmarks

- Root cause analysis for any HAPU

- Discussion of any problems identified during monthly prevalence studies and development of an action plan

- Development of nursing policies and procedures (prevention strategies, bed algorithm, wound care products, and so forth)

- Development of physician order sets to support prevention and treatment

- Sharing of unit-based pressure ulcer prevention strategies (such as elimination of cloth incontinence pads in the CICU)

Teamwork continues within and between units. On the CICU, experienced OWLs recruited other staff so that there are now OWLs on all shifts. The OWLs conduct rounds and develop individualized plans of care. OWLs also develop communication tools, including unit "OWL consult" logs and long-term wound documentation forms, to ensure that the unit's OWL team is working toward the same goals for each patient. To sustain interunit teamwork, experienced OWLs mentor and train new OWLs for other units, even assisting with daily rounds and review of care plans to help the new OWLs build their expertise.

Empowering the OWLs to influence patient outcomes has been the most exciting and rewarding part of this journey. OWLs feel accountable for HAPU prevention on their unit and they are recognized as skin care experts by their peers and physician colleagues. They have a voice in product selection, protocol development, and implementing evidence-based practice. One OWL examined the literature on the proper pH for skin care products and was successful in replacing deodorant bar soap with proper pH skin care products on all units. In addition to bringing evidence to the bedside, an experienced OWL presented her original research on pressure ulcer risk assessment at the 2009 National Magnet Conference®.

The resource nurse model also has served as an effective strategy for empowering all bedside staff. Bedside nurses understand clinical issues and will find practical and creative solutions. For example, because of the length of time CICU patients spend in the operating room and their post-operative instability, the CICU staff noted that their patients needed to be placed on the correct bed surface immediately in the operating room (OR). They arranged to take the appropriate bed to the OR suite so the patient could be transferred from the operating table directly onto the bed.

When bedside nurses observed that the existing turning wedges were unacceptable for bariatric patients, they worked with the Patient Care Value Analysis Committee to pilot several wedges and select one product for bariatric patients and another for all other patients. When staff feel a sense of ownership for their own practice and feel supported by nursing leadership, innovative ways to enhance patient outcomes flourish.

Reducing HAPUs through Frequent Data Collection

Along with the OWL resource nurse model, monthly prevalence studies have proved to be a breakthrough strategy for the PUP team. In 2006, nursing leadership implemented monthly prevalence studies and weekly rounds to more closely track and trend data. The methodical data collection process serves not only as a means to calculate HAPU rates, but also to identify problems that need to be addressed.

When the materials management group replaced sequential compression device sleeves with a different product, OWL nurses noted in the next prevalence study that the new sleeve's ridges were causing pressure-related skin breakdown. Since continual sleeve rotation was too prone to problems, the PUP team quickly requested that the former product be brought back into stock. The PUP team's request was then implemented system-wide. Similarly, the PUP team and respiratory therapists worked together to implement new facemasks for patients on continuous bi-level positive airways pressure (BiPap) after device-related pressure ulcers were noted during a prevalence study.

When a new critical care unit at Shands had a HAPU rate spike during a monthly prevalence study, the PUP team acted immediately. Experienced OWLs assisted the new unit's OWLs with plans of care and consults. The unit subsequently achieved new low rates. Frequent data collection reinforces HAPU prevention as a priority and allows for a quick response to preventable causes.

Monitoring Progress

The PUP team reviews individual unit and aggregate unit-type monthly data, using NDNQI comparison data to evaluate progress and set goals. SUF aims to consistently achieve HAPU rates below the NDNQI mean. Each unit's data with goals clearly identified are posted to communicate to all staff the progress for their patient population. Units not eligible to submit HAPU data to NDNQI still conduct monthly prevalence studies and use the most similar unit type data from NDNQI for benchmarking.

For calendar year 2006, SUF's combined adult ICU Stage II and above HAPU rate was 12.1%, higher than the NDNQI mean of 10.5% for critical care units in hospitals with over 500 beds. SUF's combined adult medical–surgical rate was 3.0%, compared with the NDNQI mean of 2.6%. By the end of 2009, the annual combined rates were 7.1% for ICUs and 1.2% for medical–surgical units, both of which were below

TABLE 1.

Annual Combined Rates of HAPUs Stage II and Above

	2006		2009	
	SUF[a]	NDNQI[b]	SUF[a]	NDNQI[b]
Unit Type				
Adult intensive care units (AICUs)	12.1	10.5	7.1	8.8
Adult medical–surgical units	3.0	2.6	1.2	2.0

Notes:

[a]Annual combined rates are the percent of all AICU or medical–surgical patients with a Stage II or above ulcer during SUF's monthly prevalence surveys. (SUF = Shands Hospital at the University of Florida)

[b]NDNQI data are the annual average unit-type means for hospitals with over 500 beds, calculated from 4Q06 and 4Q09 reports.

the NDNQI means. All of the hospital's areas have improved and are holding their gains. Table 1 summarizes the results.

CICU especially has continued to reduce pressure ulcer rates through support of its management team and the expertise of its OWL resource nurses on all shifts. Beginning in January 2007, CICU's monthly prevalence rates have been below the NDNQI mean for 31 out of 36 months. CICU achieved a Stage II and above HAPU rate of 0% for 11 out of 36 months. As illustrated in Figure 4, CICU's quarterly NDNQI rates have routinely been below the national median as well.

Costs and Benefits

Early in the pressure ulcer prevention program, nursing leadership recognized the need for bed surfaces that provided pressure redistribution for high-risk patients.

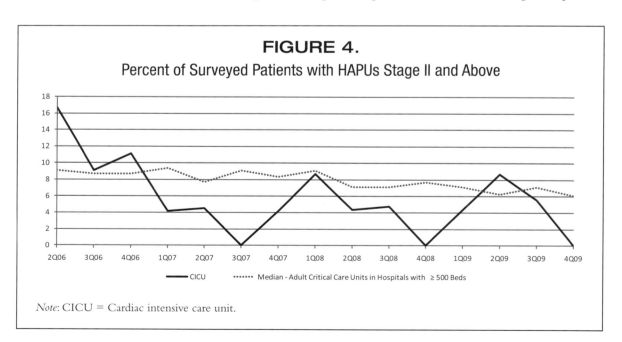

FIGURE 4.

Percent of Surveyed Patients with HAPUs Stage II and Above

Note: CICU = Cardiac intensive care unit.

NDNQI Case Studies in Nursing Quality Improvement

Since staff had been educated about the importance of using appropriate surfaces as a key intervention to prevent and treat pressure ulcers, use of rental surfaces skyrocketed in 2007. The CNSs, CWOCNs, and OWLs presented data to administration on the benefit of purchasing new low-air-loss mattresses versus continuing the use of rental surfaces. Although the cost for replacement surfaces was approximately $1 million, the cost savings for rental beds was approximately $400,000 per year. The new bed surfaces were purchased in 2008.

Paid time for staff education was another primary cost. When building the OWL program, salary dollars for education were approximately $10,000 per year. This yearly education cost will decrease for 2010 onward as only "replacement OWLs" will need initial extensive training. Salary dollars for ongoing OWL activities, such as monthly prevalence studies, weekly skin rounds, and PUP meetings, were approximately $48,000 for 2009. Overall, the program costs are approximately $60,000 per year. However, the benefits far exceed the costs.

Cost savings have been realized through improved outcomes. Not only have the total number of patients with HAPUs decreased, there has also been a reduction in the stages of ulcers. The average number of Stage III, IV, or unstageable ulcers observed during the hospital's monthly prevalence studies fell from 8.7 in 2006 to 3.7 in 2009. Since higher-stage ulcers incur higher treatment costs, this reduction in stages represents additional cost savings. As noted in the literature, the economic impact of pressure ulcer reduction initiatives is difficult to quantify precisely (Legood & McInnes, 2005; Trueman & Whitehead, 2010). The Centers for Medicare and Medicaid Services (CMS) estimate of $43,180 per patient and WOCN estimate of $50,000 per patient establishes a valid range for true costs to treat pressure ulcers (Dorner, Posthauer, & Thomas, 2009). Using the average number of patients identified during monthly prevalence studies multiplied by 12, nursing leadership estimated that to treat patients with Stage III or higher pressure ulcers, the costs to SUF ranged from $4.5–$5.2 million in 2006; $2.5–$3

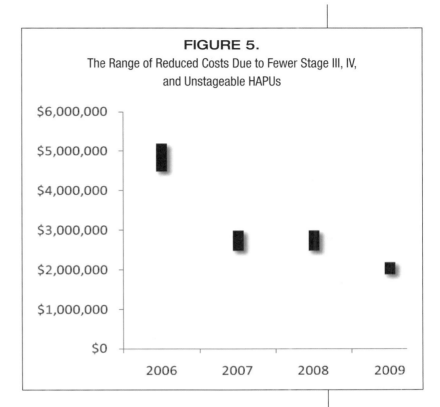

FIGURE 5.
The Range of Reduced Costs Due to Fewer Stage III, IV, and Unstageable HAPUs

million in both 2007 and 2008; and $1.9–$2.2 million in 2009. Over these four years, more than half of the costs for these patients were averted, representing a savings of over $2.5 million. Litigation costs decreased as well. Figure 5 summarizes these results.

Next Steps

The hospital's experiences over the last six years have shown that this nursing-sensitive indicator requires just as much emphasis now as when the pressure ulcer prevention program was first initiated. The data obtained through ongoing monitoring, at both weekly rounds and monthly prevalence studies, have stimulated staff to question their practice and supported a climate of evidence-based practice. Staff have engaged in nursing research studies, extensively investigated the evidence available in the literature, and changed practices when appropriate.

The PUP team continues to review data and recommend new goals annually. The action plan for HAPU prevention is never a static document. It is a dynamic process that extends from one year to the next as new issues are identified and addressed. Staff take great pride in the results obtained on this nursing-sensitive indicator as evidence of the excellent care provided by Magnet nurses at SUF.

References

Dorner, B., Posthauer, M. E., & Thomas, D. (2009). The role of nutrition in pressure ulcer prevention and treatment: National Pressure Ulcer Advisory Panel white paper. *Advances in Skin & Wound Care, 22*(5), 212–221.

Legood, R., & McInnes, E. (2005). Pressure ulcers: Guideline development and economic modeling. *Journal of Advanced Nursing, 50*(3), 307–314.

Trueman, P., & Whitehead, S. (2010). The economics of pressure-relieving surfaces: An illustrative case study of the impact of high-specification surfaces on hospital finances. *International Wound Journal, 7*(1), 48–54.

War on Wounds in the Adult Intensive Care Units

Janet Nowland, MS, RN, CWOCN
Team Leader, Wound Care Team
Janet.Nowland@sjmc.org

Jocelyn Wickey, BSN, RN
Project Specialist

St. John Medical Center
Tulsa, Oklahoma
www.sjhealthsystem.com

Case Study Highlights

The Wound Care Team's paradigm shift from treatment to prevention set the stage for improved skin assessment and preventive interventions. Point-of-care education was implemented by the new certified wound, ostomy, and continence nurse (CWOCN) to continually advance the skin care expertise of bedside nurses. Cost savings from reduced pressure ulcers justified a dedicated CWOCN for the intensive care units and the purchase of new prevention products.

Pressure Rising: Prevalence of Pressure Ulcers in the ICU

Patients in the critical care setting are generally at high risk for developing pressure ulcers. Immobility, reduced nutritional intake, and poor tissue perfusion are aspects of the ICU experience that contribute to the potential for skin breakdown. St. John Medical Center (Figure 1) reports the prevalence of hospital-acquired pressure ulcers (HAPUs) to the National Database of Nursing Quality Indicators® (NDNQI®). In 4Q07, HAPU prevalence in the Adult Intensive Care Unit (AICU) was 25%; in the Surgical Intensive Care Unit (SICU)

it was over 28%. The Neuro/Trauma Surgical Intensive Care Unit (NTSICU) opened in January 2008 with a limited number of beds. When the unit was fully open in 3Q08, HAPU prevalence on this unit reached 30%. Figure 2 profiles these three units.

Witnessing the upward trend in HAPU, the AICU focused on pressure ulcer prevention, with other units following their lead. Interventions in three primary areas led to rapid and sustained decreases in the incidence of HAPU: introduction to the philosophy and role of the Wound Care Team; changes in skin care practices; and point-of-care education for critical care nurses.

Battle Lines Drawn: Wound Care Team Reform

In late 2006, a newly hired nursing director was given oversight of the Wound Care Team (WCT). Assessing the activities of this team, she discovered that the focus was on treatment of existing wounds with no attention given to prevention. Networking within the nursing academic community, she recruited a certified wound, ostomy, and continence nurse who was

FIGURE 1.

Facility Profile

St. John Medical Center
Tulsa, Oklahoma
www.sjhealthsystem.com

Facility overview	St. John Medical Center is a full-service hospital serving Oklahoma, Arkansas, Kansas, Missouri, and Texas with a Level II Trauma Center and the only Joint Commission-Accredited Stroke Center in northeastern Oklahoma. St. John Medical Center has participated in NDNQI since 2005.
Teaching status	Teaching
Ownership status	Not-for-profit
Magnet® status	Magnet-designated in 2010
Staffed beds	567
Affiliations	University of Oklahoma Health Sciences Center Tulsa Medical Education Foundation
Awards	Oklahoma Nurses Association Excellence in the Workplace Environment Award, 2009 Goodwill Industries of Tulsa Employer of the Year, 2010 Get with the Guidelines Silver Award for Stroke Care, 2010

FIGURE 2.

Unit Profiles

Overview The Adult Intensive Care Unit (AICU) serves patients with high-acuity medical diagnoses, chiefly bacterial pneumonia, acute myocardial infarction (MI), and sepsis. The Surgical Intensive Care Unit (SICU) provides general surgical intensive care while the Neuro/Trauma Surgical Intensive Care Unit (NTSICU) specializes in neurologic and trauma intensive care.

Unit[a]	Staffed Beds	Total NHPPD[b]	Hours Supplied by RNs (%)	RNs with BSN Degree (%)	RNs with National Certification (%)	Average RN Experience (years)
AICU	22	16.4	83	46	6.3	4.5
SICU	26	13.8	85	68	25	4.5
NTSICU	22	18.9	78	64	4.6	4.5

Notes:

[a] Unit characteristics are reported at times that coincide with peak pressure ulcer incidence (4Q07 on AICU and SICU; 3Q08 on NTSICU). A survey conducted by an ICU manager in 2008 established the average amount of RN experience across all adult ICUs at 4.5 years.

[b] NHPPD = Nursing hours per patient day.

ready to facilitate a shift in paradigm from treatment to prevention.

The CWOCN was hired in August 2007 and became the Team Leader of the WCT. She began evaluating practice and establishing credibility among her peers by becoming a frequent, friendly, and helpful visitor at the bedside. She identified inconsistencies in the methods used to conduct quarterly HAPU prevalence surveys. She also assessed the need to make prevention of pressure ulcers more of a priority in the ICU setting. She began publishing monthly reports that compared the number of pressure ulcers in the AICU against house-wide occurrence based on variance reports generated by the WCT. (Members of the WCT are alerted whenever a patient has a Braden score of less than 14. If a pressure ulcer is discovered in the WCT assessment that follows, a variance report is completed.)

The major impetus for change came in July 2008 when the monthly reports published by the CWOCN revealed that 50% of pressure ulcers acquired at the hospital occurred in the AICU (Figure 3). At this time, the clinical educator for the AICU was looking for an outcomes project to meet academic requirements. The climate was ripe for change; the AICU's War on Wounds began with the CWOCN and the clinical educator leading the ranks.

On the War Path: Developing a Plan to Reduce Pressure Ulcers

The CWOCN and clinical educator observed several factors likely to have a causal relationship with the high rate of pressure ulcers in AICU:

- Skin assessments were not performed in a timely, consistent manner. Sometimes assessments were carried out at the end of shift; sometimes they were omitted.

- There was no real plan to prevent pressure ulcers; pressure ulcers were considered inevitable in this high-risk population.

- Bedside nurses were not familiar with products that could be used to prevent skin breakdown or products best suited for treatment of existing skin conditions.

- While national standards recommend Q2 hour turning as a prevention strategy, this was not being done in AICU. Specialty beds that provided continuous lateral rotation therapy (CLRT) were in use to prevent and treat pulmonary complications. Nurses believed CLRT negated the need to manually turn patients.

After a thorough literature review, the following strategies were selected to facilitate change:

- Establish time parameters for daily skin assessments.

- Implement skin care interventions to maintain intact skin.

- Implement a manual turning schedule.

- Provide formal training with point-of-care education.

- Include CWOCN in weekly interprofessional rounds.

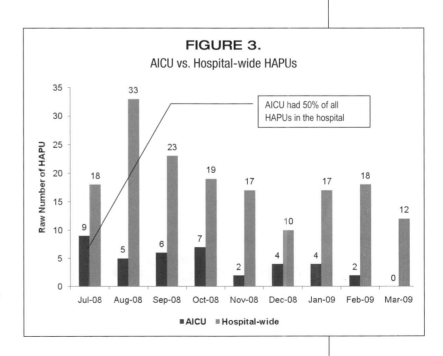

FIGURE 3.
AICU vs. Hospital-wide HAPUs

AICU had 50% of all HAPUs in the hospital

- Secure CWOCN consults early for high-risk patients.
- Initiate weekly pressure ulcer prevalence and incidence studies on the night shift until staff buy-in is secured.

The overarching goal was to reduce pressure ulcers by increasing awareness, accountability, and transparency. Specific goals were established at the patient, nurse, and facility levels respectively: maintain intact skin during a stay in AICU; perform thorough skin assessment each shift; document and report alterations in skin integrity

to CWOCN; follow turning schedule; use skin care algorithm and pressure-relieving devices; and reduce ICU-acquired pressure ulcer prevalence by 50% within six months.

Implementing the Battle Plan

The clinical educator and CWOCN developed timelines for implementation and a theme that was gender-neutral and engaged all staff. The AICU's War on Wounds was announced in this way to staff: *YOU have been called to duty. MISSION—SAVE OUR PATIENTS' SKIN.* The strategies became the "battle plan", displayed in Figure 4. Information about the War on Wounds was communicated during staff meetings and unit-based council meetings. Periodic progress reports were posted on the QI board for all to see. When the manual turning strategy was implemented, overhead announcements were made to remind staff to turn their patients.

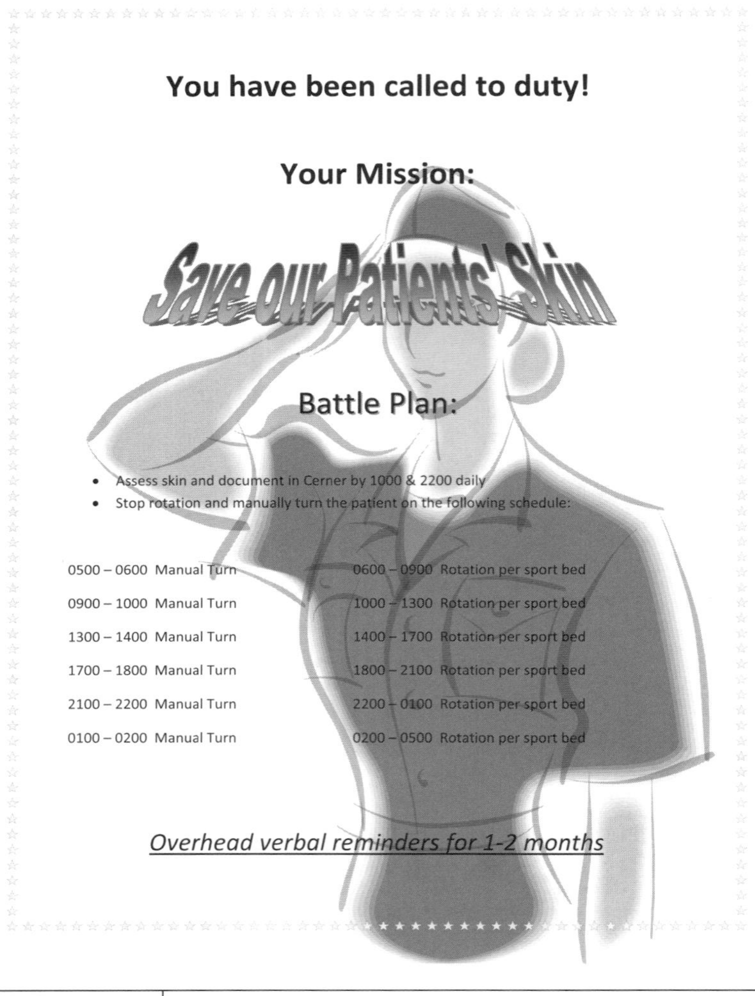

To achieve improved results, numerous processes were revised. The old and new processes are summarized in Table 1. Figure 5 presents the detailed skin care algorithm implemented to guide the selection of interventions and products.

Monitoring Progress and Making Adjustments on the Front Lines

Several procedures were used to monitor the effectiveness of these new strategies. Standardized quarterly prevalence surveys were conducted and submitted to NDNQI for benchmarking. Variance reports were completed by members of the WCT on all newly developed pressure ulcers and reviewed by key quality personnel: the quality officer, the director of the outpatient wound care center, and the director of nursing. Monthly findings based on variance reports were posted for all to see. The ICU manager was called to the bedside to inspect all pressure ulcers grown on the unit. Posting the data and engaging the manager put unit performance in the forefront, provided timely

FIGURE 4.
"Battle Plan" Poster

You have been called to duty!

Your Mission:

Save our Patients' Skin

Battle Plan:

- Assess skin and document in Cerner by 1000 & 2200 daily
- Stop rotation and manually turn the patient on the following schedule:

0500 – 0600 Manual Turn	0600 – 0900 Rotation per sport bed
0900 – 1000 Manual Turn	1000 – 1300 Rotation per sport bed
1300 – 1400 Manual Turn	1400 – 1700 Rotation per sport bed
1700 – 1800 Manual Turn	1800 – 2100 Rotation per sport bed
2100 – 2200 Manual Turn	2200 – 0100 Rotation per sport bed
0100 – 0200 Manual Turn	0200 – 0500 Rotation per sport bed

Overhead verbal reminders for 1-2 months

TABLE 1.

Old vs. New Processes

Process	Old	New
Assessment	Skin assessment performed at end of shift or not completed	Skin assessed and documented in EMR by 1000 and 2200 daily (implemented August 2008)
Turning	CLRT beds used to turn patients	Modified turning schedule combines manual turning with rotation provided by specialty beds (implemented September 2008)
Wound Care	Frequent, cost-driven changes in wound care supplies led to confusion about which product was best suited to a patient's condition	Skin care algorithm (see Figure 5) developed to guide selection of interventions and products (implemented September 2008)
	Wound care team consults limited to one encounter per referral	CWOCN began evaluating patients with wounds two to three times per week (implemented August 2008)
Education	Nursing orientation included a one-hour time slot about skin care strategies	All nurses new to adult ICUs spend 4 to 8 hours shadowing the CWOCN, focusing on risk assessment and prevention interventions (implemented Fall 2008)
	Absence of point-of-care education for staff members	Staff nurse accompanies CWOCN at patient's bedside for one-on-one sharing of expertise (implemented August 2008)
Data Collection	Prevalence and incidence studies lacked standardization	Data collection procedures were standardized and personnel received training to maximize consistency in the findings (implemented December 2007)

Note: CLRT = Continuous lateral rotation therapy; CWOCN = Certified wound, ostomy, and continence nurse; EMR = Electronic medical record; ICU = Intensive care unit.

information to the entire care team, and helped to fuel the drive to achieve improved outcomes.

New strategies were added to the War on Wounds whenever the need arose. When pressure ulcer prevalence spiked in NTSICU during 3Q08 and in SICU during 4Q08, WCT personnel were reassigned to these areas. The CWOCN became dedicated to the intensive care units, matching greatest expertise to the most vulnerable population. Additionally, with direct-care nurse feedback surrounding the inadequacy of pillows being used for manual turning, special turning wedges were purchased so that patients received optimal manual rotation while maintaining good alignment. Lastly, prevention boots were issued to patients who could not lift their heels.

Financing the Fight: Administrative Support for Pressure Ulcer Prevention

During a period of financial downturn in early 2009, nursing directors were asked to justify the existence of specialty teams such as the WCT by demonstrating that the labor expense within these entities was generating a financial return. The director of nursing practice executed a retrospective analysis based on the median cost associated with a pressure ulcer of any stage, which is approximately $21,000. Using quarterly prevalence studies to estimate annual HAPU occurrence, the director compared estimated annualized costs: $11,352,000 in 2007 versus $3,762,000 in 2008 (SMJC, 2008). This analysis garnered administrative

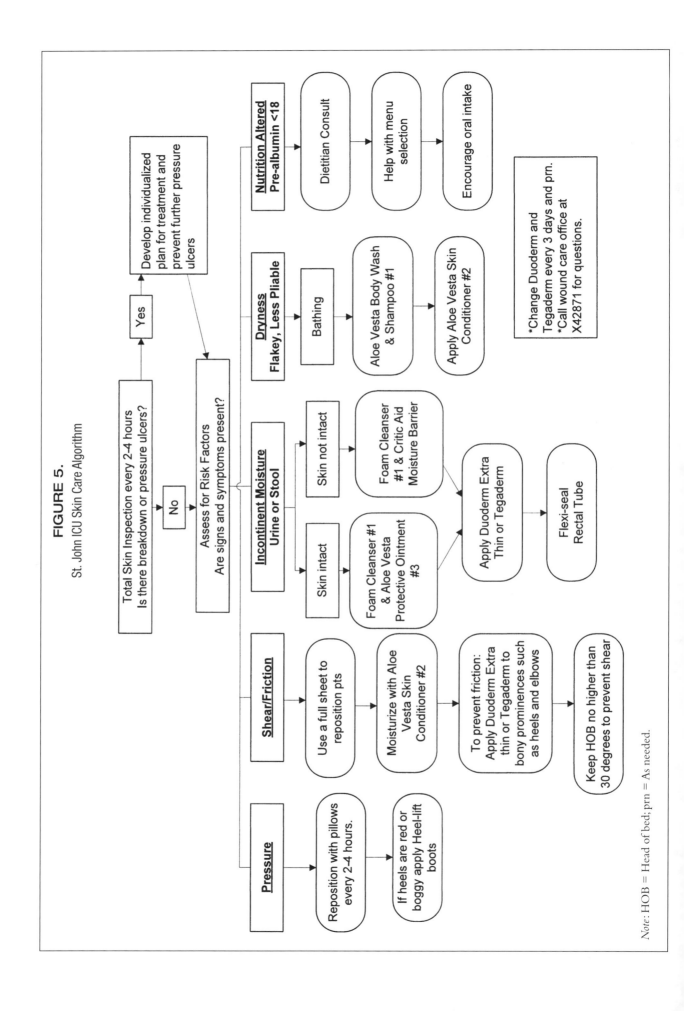

FIGURE 5.

St. John ICU Skin Care Algorithm

Total Skin Inspection every 2-4 hours
Is there breakdown or pressure ulcers?

No → Assess for Risk Factors
Are signs and symptoms present?

Yes → Develop individualized plan for treatment and prevent further pressure ulcers

Pressure
- Reposition with pillows every 2-4 hours.
- If heels are red or boggy apply Heel-lift boots

Shear/Friction
- Use a full sheet to reposition pts
- Moisturize with Aloe Vesta Skin Conditioner #2
- To prevent friction: Apply Duoderm Extra thin or Tegaderm to bony prominences such as heels and elbows
- Keep HOB no higher than 30 degrees to prevent shear

**Incontinent Moisture
Urine or Stool**
- Skin intact
  - Foam Cleanser #1 & Aloe Vesta Protective Ointment #3
- Skin not intact
  - Foam Cleanser #1 & Critic Aid Moisture Barrier
- Apply Duoderm Extra Thin or Tegaderm
- Flexi-seal Rectal Tube

**Dryness
Flakey, Less Pliable**
- Bathing
- Aloe Vesta Body Wash & Shampoo #1
- Apply Aloe Vesta Skin Conditioner #2

**Nutrition Altered
Pre-albumin <18**
- Dietitian Consult
- Help with menu selection
- Encourage oral intake

*Change Duoderm and Tegaderm every 3 days and prn.
*Call wound care office at X42871 for questions.

Note: HOB = Head of bed; prn = As needed.

36

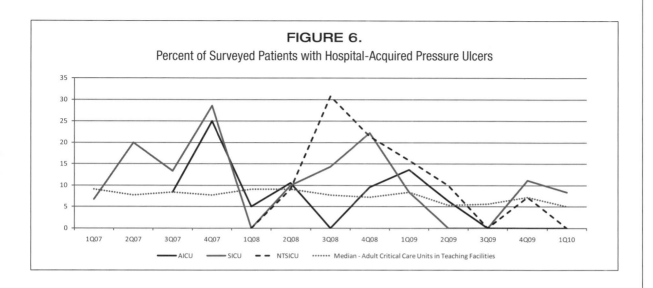

FIGURE 6.

Percent of Surveyed Patients with Hospital-Acquired Pressure Ulcers

X-axis: 1Q07, 2Q07, 3Q07, 4Q07, 1Q08, 2Q08, 3Q08, 4Q08, 1Q09, 2Q09, 3Q09, 4Q09, 1Q10

Legend: AICU — SICU — NTSICU - - - - Median - Adult Critical Care Units in Teaching Facilities

support for the WCT's efforts. The improved patient outcomes, which led to an estimated savings of $7,590,000, were tied to the ongoing availability of personnel and material resources, namely, retaining a dedicated CWOCN for adult critical care and approving the purchase of turning wedges and heel protectors.

The War on Wounds was also supported during a revision of the medical center's quality infrastructure in 2008. Strategic planning at the executive level brought about changes in the hospital's approach to quality improvement. New positions were created to oversee quality initiatives, add clarity to the reporting structure of decision-making groups, and redesign processes to improve quality and safety throughout the organization. When these changes were put into place, the CWOCN began providing monthly updates to the Quality and Safety Committee.

Victory Celebration

In AICU, improved outcomes and a sustained reduction in the incidence of HAPUs were realized over a period of 12 months. Incidence reached the 0% mark for three consecutive quarters beginning in 3Q09. NTSICU achieved a 22% incidence in HAPU (down from 30%) within the first three months after a dedicated CWOCN was assigned to adult ICUs; this downward trend continued until 0% incidence was realized 12 months after initiation. In SICU, incidence of HAPU plummeted from greater than 22% in 4Q08 to 0% by 2Q09. (See Figure 6.)

There was constant encouragement from the CWOCN, clinical educator, and manager as outcomes improved, with kudos to staff as goals were achieved. Results were posted to foster a sense of pride. Accomplishments were highlighted at several major venues: the Quality and Safety Committee, Managers and Directors, and Systems Leadership meetings. Moreover, this accomplishment has been featured at state and national conferences. With WCT reform, revised assessment and intervention guidelines, new products, improved staff education, and administrative support, the ICUs at St. John Medical Center gained a major victory in the War on Wounds.

Reference

St. John Medical Center (SJMC). 2008. Unpublished SJMC internal report, February 2008. Author: Tulsa, OK.

Comprehensive Pressure Ulcer Prevention Program Improves Outcomes for At-Risk Patients

Michael Kingan, MSN, RN, CWOCN
Clinical Specialist
Michael.J.Kingan@MedStar.net

Kathleen Srsic-Stoehr, MSN, MS, RN, NEA-BC
(Former) Senior Nursing Director, Evidence-Based Practice and Quality

Anne Marie Foley, BSc, RN
(Former) Clinical Manager/Interim Nursing Director, 2G MICU

Stefanie Lescallet, BSN, RN
Nursing Director, 2F Stroke Center Unit

Washington Hospital Center
Washington, DC
www.whcenter.org

Case Study Highlights

To reduce pressure ulcers, the Department of Nursing (DON) formed a Pressure Ulcer Performance Improvement (PI) Team, added a certified wound, ostomy, and continence nurse (CWOCN) clinical specialist, and started a Wound Resource Nurse program to increase expertise at the point of care. Individual units improved their staffing profiles, incorporated new evidence-based practices and products, and worked to create a culture that prized hospital-acquired pressure ulcer (HAPU) prevention.

Identification of the Problem

Washington Hospital Center joined NDNQI® in 2004 to benchmark pressure ulcers and other nursing indi-
cators as part of the DON quality and performance improvement plan. (See Figure 1.) In 2005, HAPU rates were above the NDNQI mean. No formalized evidence-based prevention program was in place and compliance with skin care assessment and interventions was inconsistent. This case study chronicles the DON prevention initiatives and spotlights the efforts of one critical care and one acute care medical unit in reducing HAPUs.

Development of the Department of Nursing Initiatives

In early 2006, the new DON Strategic Plan formally addressed pressure ulcer reduction targets and action plans for the first time. The Strategic Plan set three primary objectives for quality and performance improvement:

FIGURE 1.
Facility Profile

Washington Hospital Center
Washington, DC
www.whcenter.org

Facility overview   Washington Hospital Center is the largest hospital in the nation's capital, and a major referral center for complex tertiary services. The Hospital Center is a national leader in research, diagnosis, and treatment for stroke, cancer, cardiovascular, endocrine, and kidney disorders, as well as geriatric and respiratory care. The Hospital Center operates one of the country's top shock-trauma and medevac programs, and the region's only adult burn center. The hospital has participated in NDNQI since 2004.

Teaching status   Teaching

Ownership status   Private, not-for-profit

Magnet® status   Non-Magnet

Staffed beds   780 (excluding neonatal beds)

Affiliations   MedStar Health System
National Institutes of Health (NIH) Stroke Program at Washington Hospital Center Stroke Center
Numerous universities in Washington, DC, Maryland, and Virginia

Select Awards   Ranked among top hospitals in *U.S. News & World Report* for Heart and Heart Surgery (19th), Diabetes and Endocrinology (16th), and Gynecology (40th)
American Heart Association Get with the Guidelines Stroke Program Bronze Award (2008), Silver Award (2009), and Gold Award (2010)
First Washington, DC, hospital to receive the American College of Surgeons National Accreditation Program for Breast Centers and two Joint Commission Disease-Specific Care Certifications: Primary Stroke Center and Ventricular Assist Devices

FIGURE 2.
Unit Profile: 2G Medical Intensive Care Unit (MICU)

Overview   Unit 2G is a 14-bed medical intensive care unit serving patients with septicemia, intracerebral hemorrhage, cerebral occlusion, pneumonia, end-stage renal disease, and other diagnoses. The unit is the primary critical care unit for the Hospital Center's Joint Commission-certified Stroke Program. Unit 2G received the Doctors' Choice Award for commitment to the highest standards of nursing excellence and continuous quality improvement (May 2007), the Baxter Performance Improvement Award, and the American Association of Critical Care Nurses Award for Excellence in Patient Safety (May 2008).

Unit 2G	Total NHPPD	Hours Supplied by RNs (%)	Hours Supplied by Agency (%)	RNs with BSN Degree (%)	RNs with National Certification (%)	Average RN Experience (years)
2006	16.9	100	8.0	60.5	16.3	12.2
2007	15.7	100	4.3	n/r	n/r	11.7
2008	16.2	100	1.8	n/r	n/r	12.0
2009	17.3	100	2.0	73	18.8	12.0

Note: NHPPD = Nursing hours per patient day; n/r = Data not reported.

- Establish a leadership structure accountable for a culture of safety;

- Adopt evidence-based practices to improve outcomes; and

- Achieve national recognition for excellent clinical care.

The Strategic Plan also required establishing an annual target as a part of continued reduction of the HAPU rates. These targets to date are:

FY07 = NDNQI mean or better
FY08 = NDNQI mean or better
FY09 = NDNQI 50th percentile or better
FY10 = NDNQI 25th percentile or better

The DON formed the Pressure Ulcer Performance Improvement Team co-chaired by a clinical specialist and a unit director. Membership evolved to include bedside staff nurses, a physician "champion", and representatives from the hospital's Quality Resources, Risk Management, Clinical Nutrition, Physical Medicine and Rehabilitation, Clinical Resource Management, Outcomes Management, and Health Information Management departments. In 2006–2007, the PI team reviewed the literature for evidence-based prevention practices and developed targeted education programs. In addition, MedStar Health System, the parent company of Washington Hospital Center, started a system-wide task force in 2006 to provide an evidence-based practice pressure ulcer prevention and management program. Gap analysis was conducted at each hospital by interprofessional teams. The Hospital Center took the lead for MedStar in developing online prevention education modules for registered nurses (RNs), patient care technicians (PCTs), and all care providers, who completed training in late 2007.

In January 2008, a clinical specialist attended a university-based wound, ostomy, and continence nurse (WOCN) program, became certified, and began leading the WOCN service line. The WOCN consult process was incorporated into the electronic order entry system and new consult criteria were defined.

The CWOCN worked with an interprofessional team (including a physical medicine and rehabilitation specialist, a plastic surgeon, a dietician, a resource manager, and a health information management director) to revise the formulary with evidence-based wound prevention and treatment options, improve the "present on admission" identification of pressure ulcers, and conduct weekly bedside rounds.

In March 2009, to further increase expert resources, the DON implemented a unit-based wound resource nurses (WRNs) program. Based on unit size and HAPU rates, at least one bedside RN and PCT from each unit joined the WRN program for a two-year commitment. After completing specialty education, each unit's WRN team serves as a first-line, unit-based resource to their peers. WRN teams become experts in skin assessment and pressure ulcer prevention measures, including support surface and product usage and incontinence management. WRN PCTs assist in prevalence surveys and educate other PCTs about reporting mobility, nutritional intake, skin health, and incontinence problems to the patient's RN. WRN RNs assist in developing prevention plans of care, critique new products, help with implementing new policies, and evaluate unit pressure ulcer quality data.

Financial Implications of Department of Nursing Initiatives

Pressure ulcers and other adverse patient outcomes have been identified as a preventable expense for hospitals. The incremental cost of care for a patient who develops a pressure ulcer averages $15,418 and ranges from $3,529 to $59,931 (Virkstis, Matsui, Westheim, Jaggi, & Boston-Fleischhauer, 2009). Training for the clinical specialist who became a CWOCN cost $8,000. The WRN program included a one-time initial cost of $3,760. Salary costs for unit-based staff participation in the WRN training were approximately $590 per nursing unit. Additional costs included targeted education programs, application of appropriate evidence-based prevention and treatment measures, and salary expenses for WRN teams' ongoing work on their units. However, such expenses have enabled a substantial reduction of HAPU rates at the hospital, as exemplified by the critical care unit and acute care unit highlighted in this case study.

2G Medical Intensive Care Unit

Identifying the HAPU Problem and Exploring Causes

In 2006, quarterly pressure ulcer prevalence surveys on the 2G Medical Intensive Care Unit (MICU) revealed widely variable HAPU rates, which were well above the NDNQI mean. (See Figure 2.) Exploration of the causes for the high rates included structural and process issues on the unit. During the first quarter of 2006 (1Q06) when HAPU prevalence was 50%, 2G had a high staff turnover. Four temporary travel nurses were contracted to support staffing. The use of agency nurses was 11% that quarter. In addition, 2G staffing included four newly hired permanent RNs in orientation and two newly graduated RN hires in the hospital's critical care fellowship program. Staffing turbulence may have contributed to high pressure ulcer prevalence, coupled with an inconsistent knowledge and application of evidence-based practice for pressure ulcer prevention.

RNs were focused on a plan of care that addressed unstable and emergent patient conditions as the first priority; as a result, their attention may have been diverted from skin care routines for the unit's complex, critically ill patients. Although two CWOCNs were available to all nursing units for consultation, their role was primarily reactive (e.g., discussing plan of dressing care with a patient's RN). There was limited point-of-care education about prevention because of high demand for WOCN consultation services in the 750+ bed hospital.

Initiatives to Prevent HAPUs

Staffing stabilized in 2007. Agency nurse use decreased from 8% to just over 4%. The hiring of an additional

clinical manager provided sustained leadership for the unit on all shifts. Required hospital-wide online training on pressure ulcers increased nursing staff knowledge, even though some confusion still existed. During this time there was also additional education regarding the Joint Commission's National Patient Safety Goals (NPSGs) and the importance of pressure ulcer prevention. This training resulted in an overall increased awareness of proper assessment and treatment of pressure ulcers by the 2G nurses. Conversations around NPSGs became part of the daily morning report. HAPU rates decreased from an annual average of 33.6% in 2006 to an average of 21.3% in 2007. (See Figure 3.)

The hospital's WOCN clinical specialist revised the skin assessment tool to include the Braden score and a guide to various skin care products, including products to prevent and treat excoriation from urinary and fecal incontinence. This assessment tool streamlined skin care documentation onto one flowsheet and assisted nurses in selecting appropriate interventions. New skin products were introduced to the unit, including internal and external fecal containment devices that reduce the risk for skin breakdown and wound contamination. Since 2008, the use of Hill-Rom Total Care Beds has assisted with the care of clinically unstable patients with multiple risk factors for pressure ulcer development. Through an ongoing "service excellence" workgroup of nursing management and support services management, skin care product supply levels have been adjusted and response time benchmarks were established to ensure patient care supply needs were met in a timely manner.

When the hospital's plan for unit-based wound resource nurses was developed, two nurses volunteered from 2G. They continue to be extremely helpful with assessing patients and have kept the unit current on the evolution of wound care through in-services, poster presentations, and a journal club. Articles related to pressure ulcer prevention in critical care remain readily available on the unit for staff reference. The unit-based WRNs began auditing 20 medical records per month for skin assessment tool documentation compliance. Based on the audit results, RNs receive feedback with

NDNQI Case Studies in Nursing Quality Improvement

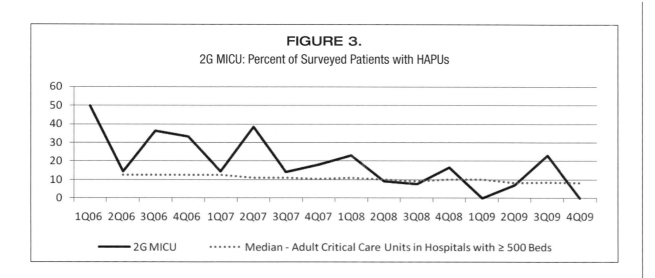

FIGURE 3.

2G MICU: Percent of Surveyed Patients with HAPUs

Legend:
——— 2G MICU ········ Median - Adult Critical Care Units in Hospitals with ≥ 500 Beds

X-axis: 1Q06 2Q06 3Q06 4Q06 1Q07 2Q07 3Q07 4Q07 1Q08 2Q08 3Q08 4Q08 1Q09 2Q09 3Q09 4Q09

additional education provided as necessary, which reinforces accountability for practice.

Monitoring Progress

The downward trend in HAPU prevalence on 2G coincided with the multiple improvements in staffing, pressure ulcer education and awareness, new products, a revised assessment tool, and WRN bedside expertise. The annual average HAPU rate dropped to 14.1% in 2008 and 12.9% in 2009. Quarterly rates reached below the NDNQI median and zero prevalence was achieved in 1Q09 and 4Q09. The occasional elevated rate (e.g., 3Q09) may be due to the severe illnesses and multiple co-morbidities of 2G patients.

Celebrating Success and Continuing the Work

Consistent staffing, education about evidence-based practices, and use of the Braden risk assessment scale to assist in a specific plan of care have resulted in a culture change. Staff now believe that skin care to prevent and manage pressure ulcers can be incorporated into the complex care of unstable, critically ill patients. The unit celebrates its reduced HAPU rates at staff meetings, interprofessional rounds, and PI huddles.

Maintaining improved patient outcomes is an ongoing effort and there is always room for improvement. Supporting the role of the WRNs through their development as members of the hospital's pressure ulcer PI team is essential. These unit-based nurses will continue to develop expertise to ensure appropriate assessment, intervention, and staff support. Staff on 2G will soon be involved in evaluating a new support surface and will continue staff education and accountability for further reduction in pressure ulcers.

2F Stroke Center/Medical Unit

Identifying the HAPU Problem and Exploring Causes

In 2006, HAPU prevalence rates for the 2F Stroke Center/Medical Unit were above the NDNQI mean. (See Figure 4.) The unit's average rate in 2006 was 14.9%, with a mean of 22.6% for Q106 and Q206 and 7.28% for Q306 and Q406. At this time, a new unit nursing director along with three clinical managers came on board and recognized the problem. The staff lacked knowledge about evidence-based prevention practices and needed to view pressure ulcers as preventable for patients with deficits, such as paralysis, ventilator dependency, and decreased mobility. Pressure ulcers had been recognized as a reactive problem with consults to the WOCN service used to manage a patient with a pressure ulcer.

FIGURE 4.
Unit Profile: 2F Stroke Center/Medical Unit

Overview Unit 2F is a 30-bed adult medical unit primarily serving patients diagnosed with hemorrhagic or occlusive type stroke. The unit is the primary acute care unit for the Hospital Center's Joint Commission-certified Stroke Program. Unit 2F received the Doctors' Choice Award for commitment to the highest standards of nursing excellence and continuous quality improvement (May 2008).

Unit 2F	Total NHPPD	Hours Supplied by RNs (%)	Hours Supplied by LPNs (%)	Hours Supplied by PCTs (%)	RNs with BSN Degree (%)	RNs with National Certification (%)	Average RN Experience (years)
2006	7.6	64.5	14.5	21	38	3.9	11
2007	7.4	64.5	14.0	21	n/r	1.9	10
2008	8.1	61.3	14.3	24.5	n/r	3.4	10
2009	8.4	69	0	28.5	55	3.3	12

Note: NHPPD = Nursing hours per patient day; LPN = Licensed practical nurse; n/r = Data not reported.

The staffing skill mix was not ideal, particularly regarding enough support staff to assist with turning of patients. At this time, interventions based on Braden risk assessments were not being carried out as a proactive measure and assessment scores were inconsistent. The use of moisture-retaining items, such as disposable underpads and adult disposable briefs, were also thought to play a role in the number of HAPUs.

Initiatives to Prevent HAPUs

In 2007, the unit's nursing director involved nursing staff in the conduct of prevalence surveys and auditing patient assessment flow sheets. Skin integrity assessments or reassessments were conducted every shift. Documentation audits were conducted on patients with Braden scores ≤ 18.

The use of moisture-retaining materials was decreased or eliminated in early 2007; disposable underpads were completely eliminated and use of adult disposable briefs was decreased. For patients with incontinence and Braden scores ≤ 18, the plan of care was to limit layers of linen and incorporate barrier cream application for prevention or treatment measures. Following this change, HAPUs were at 0% for four consecutive quarters. This 2F initiative also resulted in a supply cost saving to the unit with the reduction of disposable products.

In 2Q08, an increase in HAPUs occurred on the unit. A more focused and structured rounding strategy was implemented throughout all units in the Department of Nursing. Patient rounding on the unit increased from every two hours to every hour, addressing elimination needs, turning, pain assessment, and any other specific patient need. PCTs were added in 2008 and 2009 to assist with activities of daily living (ADLs), turning, and identifying patients at risk for pressure ulcers. In 2009, a reduction in force of five LPNs with replacement in RN positions enhanced the RN and PCT team accountability for pressure ulcer risk identification, prevention, and intervention measures.

From 2006 to the present, various education and communication strategies have been implemented to increase staff awareness, knowledge, and feedback for accountability. Communication strategies on 2F included shift handoff huddles, monthly and weekly staff meetings with feedback on wound assessment audits, visual aids posted on the unit, debriefings with nursing staff on specific patient problems, and the completion of HAPU occurrence reports with defined corrective actions for resolution. Since 2009, the unit's wound resource RN and PCT have been mentors and resources for their peers, providing wound monitoring data feedback, guiding staff on proper procedures with specific at-risk patients, and updating staff based on the monthly prevention education WRN teams receive.

NDNQI Case Studies in Nursing Quality Improvement

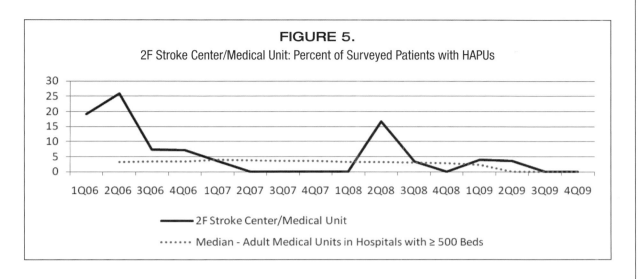

FIGURE 5.

2F Stroke Center/Medical Unit: Percent of Surveyed Patients with HAPUs

——— 2F Stroke Center/Medical Unit

······· Median - Adult Medical Units in Hospitals with ≥ 500 Beds

Monitoring Progress

A decrease in pressure ulcer rates began in 2007 with only a 3.5% rate in 1Q07 and 0% in the four subsequent quarters. After the spike in 2Q08, rates returned again to below the NDNQI median and reached 0% for three of the last five quarters. (See Figure 5.)

Celebrating Success and Continuing the Work

Announcements and celebrations of positive patient outcomes and staff accomplishments are conducted during staff meetings. RNs and PCTs can now specify a plan of care for patients at risk for HAPUs. The unit WRN program has provided point-of-care expertise. Feedback on random audits for present-on-admission documentation compliance, Braden risk assessments, and preventive plans of care have increased staff knowledge and improved patient care. Two clinical managers' positions have been converted to clinical care facilitator positions to improve unit-based coordination of care and further improve patient outcomes. Through frequent patient rounds, ongoing prevention processes, and the expertise of the WRN team, Unit 2F will continue to work toward zero tolerance for pressure ulcers.

Ongoing Pressure Ulcer Prevention Program

DON and unit-level improvements led to substantial decreases in HAPU prevalence at Washington Hospital Center. To sustain this improvement, HAPU prevention activities are ongoing. Recently, the DON worked with the shared governance Practice Council to develop and pilot test a new wound prevention and treatment protocol for house-wide implementation in 2010. New criteria were also developed for support surface selection to ensure correct surface selection while managing costs. The DON recently conducted a business case analysis to broaden WOCN services and achieve revenue generation through improved patient outcomes. Workshops and journal clubs continue to expand staff's application of evidence-based prevention techniques while competency-based validation and revised shift-to-shift communication methods focus accountability on practice. Achieving success is incremental and ongoing prevention efforts are required to attain progressive, consistent, and sustained optimal patient outcomes across all patient care areas.

Reference

Virkstis, K. L., Matsui, P. N., Westheim, J., Jaggi, T., & Boston-Fleischhauer, C. (2009). Safeguarding quality: Building the business case to prevent nursing-sensitive hospital-acquired conditions. *Journal of Nursing Administration, 39*(7/8), 350–355.

Incremental Changes in Culture, Workforce, and Products Reduce Hospital-Acquired Pressure Ulcers in the Intensive Care Setting

Barbara Twombly, BSN, RN, WOCN
Intensive Care Wound Care Nurse
Twombly.Barbara@scrippshealth.org

Amy Stuck, MSN, RN
Intensive Care Unit Advanced Practice Nurse

Kathleen Blechertas, PT, WCC
Manager, Physical Therapy

Kathleen Reilly, BSN, RN
Project Manager, Performance Improvement

Nathan Dollick, BSN, RN, CCRN
Patient Care Manager, SICU

Scripps Memorial Hospital, La Jolla
La Jolla, California
www.scripps.org

Case Study Highlights

Structural changes (e.g., unit redesign, fewer agency nurses) preceded numerous practice changes focused on creating a culture of prevention. With persistent incremental interventions targeting unit culture, workforce, products, and staff education, annual hospital-acquired pressure ulcer (HAPU) rates fell from over 20% to under 7% on the surgical intensive care unit.

Overview of Pressure Ulcer Prevention Efforts

HAPU rates in the intensive care units at Scripps Memorial Hospital, La Jolla (SMH-LJ), were near the 90th percentile for NDNQI® and the Collaborative Alliance for Nursing Outcomes (CalNOC) in 2005 and 2006. The Chief Nurse Executive, Chief Financial Officer, and Performance Improvement Director worked to develop a strategic plan to address the unit structure and workforce issues that were contributing to high HAPU rates. Subsequently, a series of changes in daily practice were used to promote a culture of HAPU prevention. With continual practice and workforce and product improvements, HAPU rates have successfully been reduced. (See Figure 1.)

Structural Changes Pave the Way for Improvement

Before April 2007, the intensive care units at SMH-LJ were considered one unit, led by one manager who oversaw 41 beds and more than 120 employees. The manager's effectiveness was limited by a large span of control covering multiple, geographically separate units. This management structure did not allow for clear communication of expectations or realistic monitoring for accountability. Even though data on hospital-acquired pressure ulcers were available and communicated to staff, several factors contributed to the challenge of reducing pressure ulcers in the units. First, 30% of the intensive care unit (ICU) nurses were contracted travelers who had little organizational understanding, buy-in, or accountability. Second, experienced core nurses were taxed with frequently orienting the incoming traveler staff. Additionally,

expert wound nurse resources were limited. Finally, the staff in the ICU did not consider skin integrity a priority in the critically ill patient and often perceived pressure ulcers as unavoidable.

Despite several approaches taken to decrease the rate of pressure ulcers in the ICU, the rates were not improving. Hospital administration reviewed the HAPU data, met with the manager and staff, who together developed a strategic plan to make improvements in the ICU. Four key areas were targeted for change.

Unit Design:

The intensive care unit was separated into three specialty units in the spring of 2007 and two additional managers were hired. This improved managerial effectiveness and increased staff expertise for a specific patient population.

Workforce:

In order to eliminate the use of travelers, administration made a commitment to hire Student Nurse Externs (SNEs) with the expectation that a majority of these students would remain with SMH-LJ after graduation. SNEs are baccalaureate senior nursing students who participate in a work study program under the guidance and preceptorship of a critical care RN. Additionally, managers in the medical-surgical areas were instructed to over-hire RNs by 20% with the understanding that they would be "feeder" units for the ICU intern training program. The intern training program, previously offered annually, was increased to quarterly and the number of RNs accepted for each training session was doubled. To assist staff nurses with reducing pressure ulcers, an ICU Wound Care Nurse was hired two days per week. The Wound Care Nurse initiated "Wound Wednesdays" to evaluate and update skin care plans with each patient's primary RN.

Education:

Wound care guidelines were formulated and reviewed with each nurse and placed in every bedside chart. Mandatory basic wound care classes were instituted for all new nursing employees.

Products:

Pressure redistribution mattresses were purchased for all ICU beds.

Causes of HAPU Further Explored

Despite the changes initiated prior to 2007, the annual HAPU rate only decreased from 21.6% to 19.7%, still above the NDNQI mean for comparable hospitals. It was determined that a more focused, in-depth analysis was needed. Over the next two years, the Critical Care Advanced Practice Nurse, ICU Wound Care Nurse, and a representative from Performance Improvement compared HAPU rates to national and state benchmarks, scrutinized data about the locations and stages of wounds, and looked for patterns in wounds associated with medical devices, long procedure times, or inadequate nutrition. In addition, a root cause analysis was conducted on two complex cases. From this analysis, several root causes were uncovered:

- Lack of staff accountability for outcomes, compounded by the remaining number of travelers

(16%) and an increasing volume of novice nurses from the intern training program

- Lack of a standardized approach to skin assessment

- Inconsistent knowledge about the implications of impaired skin integrity

- Braden scale and subscale scores were not used as triggers for interventions

Analysis of prevalence data and root causes led to a series of systematic rapid improvement cycles using the Plan-Do-Check-Act (PDCA) model, which concentrated on culture, workforce, products, and education. Improvements were aimed at accomplishing two goals: Decrease Stage II or greater pressure ulcers in the ICU to below the NDNQI mean for similar units in similar hospitals, and eliminate device-related pressure ulcers (wounds due to cervical collars, oxygen tubing, nasogastric [NG] tubes, bi-level positive airway pressure [BiPAP] masks, neck braces, pneumatic compression devices, and so on). SMH-LJ's three critical care units experienced variations in success in changing culture and outcomes, as units evaluated their own data to identify their specific trends and needs. The Surgical Intensive Care Unit (SICU) demonstrated the most consistent and dramatic improvement and will therefore be highlighted in this case study. From a high of 33.3%, the unit experienced progressively more quarters with fewer than 10% Stage II HAPU. By 2009, the SICU's annual rate declined to 6.6%. (See Figures 2 and 3.)

Addressing Culture

To create a unit culture where HAPU prevention and skin integrity were valued, multiple small changes were instituted beginning in 2007, including changes in risk assessment, daily rounds, and HAPU data monitoring. In the area of risk assessment, staff surveys and audits revealed inconsistency in completing the Braden scale and linking the score to the plan of care. Staff indicated that completing the Braden scale had become a labor-intensive "task" versus a useful tool. In an effort to simplify the process and gain compliance, a brief risk assessment was created that placed all patients at "high

FIGURE 2.
Unit Profile

Overview The Surgical Intensive Care Unit (SICU) serves a post-surgical and trauma patient population. SICU is a recipient of the AACN Beacon Award for Excellence.

Unit	Staffed Beds	Total NHPPD	Hours Supplied by RNs (%)	RNs with BSN Degree (%)	RNs with National Certification (%)	Average RN Experience (years)
SICU	12	18.7	100	76	48	11

Note: NHPPD = Nursing hours per patient day.

risk" or "extreme high risk", then linked the risk level directly to the Patient Management Tool (plan of care). Patients labeled as "extreme high risk" would receive increased frequency of skin assessment and turning, optimized nutrition regimen, and an evaluation for appropriate bed surface to prevent pressure injury.

Assessment of skin integrity was added to daily inter-professional rounds led by an advance practice nurse and an intensivist. In addition, daily skin rounds by the unit manager or charge nurse began to promote accountability and reinforce expectations for skin assessment. Skin care was discussed at five-minute shift stand up meetings and reinforced as a priority on the "Daily Goals" sheet. Changes in data monitoring further served to encourage accountability. HAPU prevalence studies were increased from quarterly to monthly, with monthly rates posted on the unit.

In 2008, the SICU had a change in management. The new manager was highly motivated and enthusiastic to keep the momentum going for preventing HAPUs. The

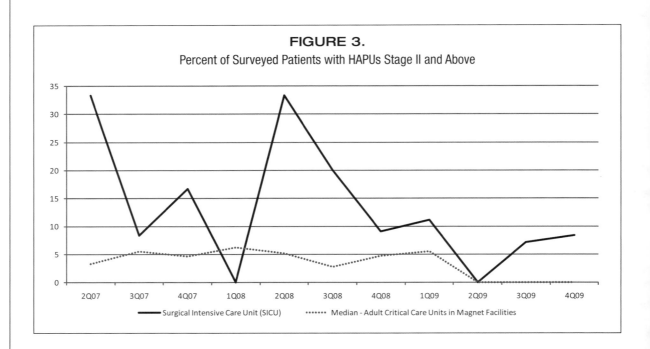

FIGURE 3.
Percent of Surveyed Patients with HAPUs Stage II and Above

Legend: Surgical Intensive Care Unit (SICU) — Median - Adult Critical Care Units in Magnet Facilities

manager reinforced expectations for unit performance below the mean rate of Stage II or greater HAPUs in NDNQI Magnet® hospitals, directed charge nurses to meet with each patient's bedside nurse daily to conduct visual skin checks and review risk assessments and interventions, and began presenting case studies at staff meetings to discuss best practices in skin care.

The manager also started "On Your Watch", a process of notifying the bedside RNs when a pressure ulcer developed during their shift. The program was intended to elicit suggestions for pressure ulcer prevention. However, when the manager determined the program was perceived negatively by unit staff, a more positive approach to accountability was selected. Beginning in 2009, pizza parties were held to celebrate successful discharge of long-term, high-risk patients without a HAPU.

Transforming a unit culture requires a persistent, multi-faceted effort. In 2009, a number of changes continued to promote a culture of accountability for skin integrity. Shift change skin assessments were initiated and performed in tandem by on-going and off-going nurses. Annual job performance standards were modified to include unit-based goals determined by NDNQI benchmarks. For six months, weekly prevalence studies were used to gather more robust data on unit-based HAPUs. Finally, the hospital's Interdisciplinary Quality Council sanctioned the creation of a HAPU Task Force to evaluate processes and create a streamlined approach to risk assessment and pressure ulcer prevention.

Workforce Continuity and Specific Roles

By 2009, the SICU significantly reduced its traveler usage to less than 1%. Also, turnover decreased from 13% to 6%, nearing the strategic goal set prior to 2007. To further support pressure ulcer reduction, two additional workforce changes were made. The existing lift team was expanded to accommodate an every-two-hour turning schedule in the SICU for high-risk,

heavy-lift patients. When the Wound Care Nurse resigned her position, an ICU Clinical Mentor who was Wound Care Certified (WCC) assumed the role and is currently being funded by the hospital to obtain her Wound, Ostomy, and Continence Nurse (WOCN) certification.

Products for Preventing Skin Breakdown

A succession of new products, along with policy changes related to the use of medical devices, has contributed to fewer pressure ulcers. Product and policy changes were made whenever a need was revealed from analysis of prevalence data and root causes. In 2008, the SICU responded to a growing number of suspected deep tissue injuries on nares by altering the standard of care to require repositioning of NG tubes every 24 hours. Staff nurses are currently involved in a county-wide Evidence-Based Practice Consortium that is investigating the best method to secure nasal tubes to prevent skin breakdown. A new policy also requires an RN to be in attendance to assess skin condition when endotracheal (ET) tubes are repositioned or re-taped.

In 2009, three new devices were put into practice. Preventative Mepilex Lite Dressings were placed under BiPAP masks in response to a number of pressure ulcers noted on the face, on the bridge of the nose, and above the ears of patients with BiPAP masks. Initially these wounds did not decrease, so the WCC nurse conducted classes for the respiratory care professionals which drastically decreased the occurrence of these pressure injuries. Occian backs were added to the Aspen cervical collars in response to a high number of occipital ulcers on trauma patients. These ulcers were all but eliminated within 6 months. Lastly, the SICU instituted the use of indwelling fecal containment devices to decrease moisture-related skin damage for incontinent patients.

To address pressure ulcer risk occurring outside the ICU, pressure-reducing surfaces in the emergency department (ED) and operating room (OR) were examined. In 2008, a new policy required that patients expected to remain in the ED for more than two hours be transferred from a gurney to a pressure-reducing bed. In 2009, the Wound Care Nurse collaborated with surgical staff to upgrade surfaces in the surgery department. Based on an increase in HAPUs on foreheads of patients who were prone during surgery, the size of pressure-reducing surfaces in the operating room was modified.

Continuing Staff Education

Beyond the staff education that occurred during the culture and product improvements, and the education routinely provided by the ICU Wound Care Nurse, targeted staff education continued throughout 2009. Scripps Health rolled out a system-wide campaign to "See Pink . . . Think" in order to increase awareness and communication, improve risk assessment, and promote patient and family participation in pressure ulcer prevention. The HAPU Task Force created Skin Assessment Man (SAM) to promote a standardized approach to skin assessment and to provide a tool for bedside education and annual competency evaluation. The task force focused education using SAM for the OR and ED.

In 2009, the Braden Scale was reinstituted in conjunction with re-education for the roll out of a system-wide electronic medical record. The hospital is in the process of bundling interventions based on patients' Braden Scale and subscale scores and linking these to the plan of care.

Costs and Benefits

While measuring the precise fiscal impact of all the changes implemented is beyond the scope of this case study, the benefits have far outweighed the costs. In general, new products had a mixed financial impact, in some instances costing more and in other instances producing savings. Reducing managerial span of con-

trol, over-hiring RNs, and expanding use of student externs were all expensive changes. However, in addition to decreased HAPUs, other negative outcomes were reduced in conjunction with more stable staffing, such as decreases in catheter-associated urinary tract infections, central line-associated blood stream infections, and use of restraints. Nurse, patient, and physician satisfaction scores improved and RN turnover rates decreased. All of these have a corresponding fiscal benefit. The changes resulted in improved patient care and better work environments, with an overall decrease in hospital costs.

Lessons Learned

Without the backing of senior leadership, including the structural changes and the pledge to secure a more stable staff, the effect on outcomes would have been limited. Initially, the frequent adjustments to skin care policies and procedures were met with resistance, but once outcomes began to improve and SICU nurses were no longer overwhelmed with orienting travelers, the changes were accepted more readily. When initiating these changes, it was essential to communicate the rationale and the positive implications for patients. The passion of the frontline manager and the critical care wound nurses fueled the commitment to an ultimate goal of "zero" HAPU. Staff know their HAPU rates, they know who is at risk, and there is a palpable pride in decreasing the prevalence of pressure ulcers.

The reduction in HAPU rate required interprofessional, multi-level interventions. Over the past few years, numerous opportunities were identified that led to changes in unit design, management span of control, unit culture, workforce, products, and education. Initially, changes were retrospectively based on isolated occurrences discovered through individual root cause analysis. When the units separated, each with its own manager, this approach initially worked well. It allowed each individual unit to address population-specific issues. Now a systematic approach promotes needed changes in care processes. By focusing on global trends while sharing and incorporating population-specific challenges, the hospital has come together to further reduce or eliminate HAPUs. Today, the focus is to proactively identify all areas of potential skin risk and implement comprehensive prevention and intervention strategies.

The journey toward improvement has been incremental, with each change contributing to the overall progress. Expert clinicians, bedside staff, and leadership were all essential to the success of the improvement effort. The team was fortunate to have the support of all the aforementioned groups combined with a passion for reducing patient injury. It is an honor to share this story and to hopefully inspire others to be persistent, fearless to make change, and dedicated to quality patient care.

Weekly Falls Review Team: Nurse-Driven Interprofessional Initiative to Decrease Patient Falls in the Acute Care Setting

Patricia G. Shaffer, MSN, JD, RN
Director, Professional Nursing Practice
patti.shaffer@christushealth.org

CHRISTUS St. Michael Health System
Texarkana, Texas
www.christusstmichael.org

Case Study Highlights

Implementation of a Falls Prevention Protocol, online falls education for all hospital associates, inception of an interprofessional Weekly Falls Review Team, and purchase of fall prevention equipment resulted in a reduction in total inpatient falls.

Addressing the Problem of Patient Falls

Since the Institute of Medicine released *To Err is Human: Building Safer Heath Systems* (IOM, 2000), patient safety has become of paramount importance to many hospitals and national quality organizations. According to the Institute for Healthcare Improvement (IHI), patient falls are one of the most common occurrences reported in hospitals (IHI, 2010). In 2005, the Joint Commission's *National Patient Safety Goals for Hospitals* added an initiative to reduce the risk of patient harm resulting from falls (Geller & Guzman, 2005). In October 2008, the Centers for Medicare and Medicaid Services (CMS) discontinued reimbursement for eight hospital-acquired conditions; costs related to patient injuries from falls are no longer paid (CMS, 2007). This national focus on reducing patient falls has engendered a climate of change in individual hospitals and health systems.

In the spring of 2007, the CHRISTUS Health Chief Nurse Executive (CNE) Council met to determine how best practices could be implemented throughout the CHRISTUS Health System. As a result, the CHRISTUS Health Evidence-Based Advisory Council was established, with one nursing director from each of the system's regions serving on the council. Due in part to the prevalence of falls throughout the CHRISTUS Health System, developing a fall prevention protocol became the focus of the Evidence-Based Advisory Council's first face-to-face meeting in July 2007. Over the next several months the Council met bi-weekly via teleconference to conduct literature searches, summarize the evidence, and translate the evidence into a universally applicable protocol that could be implemented system-wide to reduce patient falls and associated costs. An initial goal was set for each CHRISTUS Health hospital to achieve at least an 8% reduction in the raw number of falls from the previous year. As part of the CHRISTUS Health System, the CHRISTUS

FIGURE 1.
Facility Profile

CHRISTUS St. Michael Health System
Texarkana, Texas
www.christusstmichael.org

Facility overview	Centrally located in northeast Texas just off I-30, CHRISTUS St. Michael Health System serves residents of Arkansas, Texas, Louisiana, and Oklahoma. CHRISTUS St. Michael has participated in NDNQI since 2007.
Teaching status	Non-teaching
Ownership status	Not-for-profit
Magnet® status	Application submitted April 2010
Staffed beds	312
Affiliations	CHRISTUS Health
Awards	Joint Commission-certified Primary Stroke Center, 2010 Blue Distinction Center for joint replacement and cardiac care Aetna Institute of Quality Cardiac Care *Modern Healthcare* Best Places to Work in U.S., 2008 (7th) and 2009 (3rd) Ranked 6th Best Company to Work for in Texas, 2005–2010

St. Michael (CSM) nursing units (see Figures 1 and 2) embraced the system-wide fall reduction initiative.

Roll Out of the Falls Prevention Protocol

In the spring of 2008, the orthopedic unit at CSM, along with two other units in CHRISTUS Health hospitals, began piloting the newly developed protocol. Nursing staff on the pilot units were educated about the protocol through online modules. With input from the pilot units, the protocol was revised and tailored to each hospital's needs while maintaining the integrity of the protocol's evidence-based practices. Following the three-month pilot, the falls prevention protocol was rolled out to all inpatient nursing units at CSM. Every CSM associate completed the online educa-

FIGURE 2.
Unit Profiles

Overview This case study highlights improvements on six medical and/or surgical units, which serve a variety of adult patient populations.

Unit Type	Specialty	Staffed Beds	Total NHPPD	Hours Supplied by RNs (%)	RNs with BSN Degree (%)	RNs with National Certification (%)
Medical	General medicine	36	7.5	36.5	6.4	17.4
Surgical	Orthopedics	36	7.9	37.4	10.0	59.8
	General surgery	36	7.4	35.8	0	14.4
	Gynecology	20	8.5	60.3	39.4	54.1
Medical–surgical	Telemetry	31	8.3	43.3	15.8	16.0
	Stroke, telemetry	34	8.5	44.3	23.1	6.1

Note: NHPPD = Nursing hours per patient day.

tional module entitled *Falls Prevention Protocol and the Management of the Patient at Risk for Falls.*

The falls prevention protocol implemented several new processes in addition to reviving some old ones. Upon admission, transfer, or change in status, and following a fall, patients are assessed according to the Morse Fall Risk Screening Assessment. Fall prevention strategies are implemented according to the patient's score. Patients at moderate or high risk for falls are identified with a yellow wristband. The door to a moderate- or high-risk patient's room is identified with a yellow "dot" magnet, and with a yellow "star" if the patient has previously experienced a fall. Nurses use the Environmental Rounds for Patient Safety Checklist to conduct hourly rounds that include the 4 Ps (Position, Pain, Potty, and Pause), ensuring the patient's bed is in the low position, activating the bed alarm before leaving the room, and reminding the patient and family to call for assistance in getting out of bed.

The Weekly Falls Review Team

By October 2008, there did not seem to be an appreciable decrease in patient falls despite the implementation of the evidence-based falls prevention protocol. The existing Falls Committee at CSM met to brainstorm what else could be done. Another committee at CSM had successfully reduced length of stay by instituting weekly review of every case in which patients were hospitalized longer than five days. The Falls Committee asked themselves, "Why can't we meet every week as well, to review every patient fall?" Thus CSM established an interprofessional Weekly Falls Review Team, whose purpose is to discuss every patient fall in order to identify preventable causes of falls. A direct-care nurse chairs the team and the Director of Professional Nursing Practice serves as facilitator. Team members include the Chief Nurse Executive, Risk Management Manager, Nursing Informatics Coordinator, Nursing Staffing Resources Manager, Clinical Education Coordinator, Pharmacy Manager, Plant Operations Manager, an Occupational Therapy associate, a Quality associate, and the Housekeeping

Team Leader. Additionally, the nursing unit manager and direct-care nurse involved in each fall participate in the weekly review meeting.

At team meetings, the patient's nurse presents the patient's history, fall risk assessment, implementation of fall prevention strategies as outlined in the CHRISTUS falls prevention protocol, the events surrounding the fall, and any barriers to fall prevention. The Pharmacy Manager reviews medications received by the patient to determine any fall correlation. The Plant Operations Manager examines the functionality of fall beds, alarms, and other patient equipment. Staffing effectiveness is evaluated, as is the extent of patient and family fall prevention education.

As the team began its analysis of the circumstances surrounding patient falls, commonalities began to surface. The team determined that falls often occurred after a family member left the patient's room without letting staff know the patient was now unattended. The team reinforced the need to educate patients and families about falls prevention, and nursing staff began to request that family members tell the nurse when they leave a patient unattended. This allows the nurse to ensure the bed alarm is activated and functional. While not every patient or family member is cooperative, understanding that they or their loved one is at high risk for falls has convinced most that the nursing staff is concerned for the patient's safety.

Other commonalities identified by the team led to improvements in both accountability of nurses and implementation of additional fall prevention strategies, including never leaving a patient at high risk for falls unattended in the bathroom. The reviews also identified patient care equipment that was inadequate to meet the patient's fall prevention needs (for example, bed alarms that did not signal movement either because the patient did not weigh enough to trigger the alarm or because the alarm was simply not working).

Following the implementation of the Weekly Falls Review Team, CHRISTUS St. Michael also implemented a Falls Patient Care Profile form and a Post-

Fall Response Review form. At the time a patient fall is identified, the Falls Response Team is activated using the hospital paging console. The Rapid Response Nurse on duty, the House Supervisor, and the Unit Manager assist the patient's nurse in post-fall care, which includes thorough assessment for injuries, mental status changes, range of motion, and potential contributing factors such as orthostatic hypotension and blood glucose level. Data compiled from the Post-Fall Response Review forms revealed approximately two-thirds of patients who fell were over 60 years old and the majority of patients were alert and oriented before falling.

Acquisition of Fall Prevention Equipment

New equipment was purchased in support of the Falls Prevention initiative. Thirteen low beds and 15 Stryker fall beds were acquired with grant funds from the CHRISTUS Health System Emerald Innovations Program and with capital budget dollars respectively. The Weekly Falls Review Team identified the need to enhance the sensitivity of existing bed alarms with the purchase of conversion kits that work with the older bed inventory.

To address the needs of the high fall risk patient who is able to sit in a chair, the team proposed the purchase of additional chair pad alarms. With operational budget dollars, eight chair pad alarms were initially purchased for two nursing units that had a high number of patient falls from chairs. Ultimately, the team determined this should be available to patients on all nursing units throughout the hospital and internal grant money purchased 24 additional chair pad alarms.

Since there are often more patients at high risk for falls than there are rooms near the nurses' station, the team determined that 24 rooms throughout the various nursing units would benefit from surveillance cameras, and grant money was used for their purchase. Finally, in order to eliminate the cause of some falls during the use of bedside commodes, the team proposed the

purchase of bedside commodes with drop sides to ease patient movement onto the equipment.

Monitoring Progress

Falls are compiled with raw numbers each month and reported to each unit, the monthly Falls Committee meeting, and the monthly Safety Committee meeting. The raw number of monthly falls hospital-wide began to decrease immediately after creation of the Weekly Falls Review Team: from 28 in October 2008 to 18 in November 2008 and to 11 by May 2009. (See Figure 3.)

Falls are also reported to NDNQI® for quarterly comparison to similar hospitals. Especially notable success was achieved on the medical unit, whose total fall rate hovered around the 75th percentile prior to 3Q08 but dropped below the 25th percentile for medical units in NDNQI non-teaching hospitals by 2Q09. (See Figures 4A, 4B, and 4C.)

Although success seemed almost instantaneous, the true measure of success will be in maintaining a low patient fall rate. When the raw number of falls spiked in July and August 2009, the team identified the need for periodic educational reinforcement of the falls prevention protocol, especially for new graduates who recently completed an orientation period and have just begun practicing independently.

Celebration and Replication of Success

The Weekly Falls Review Team recognizes nursing units that demonstrate effective fall prevention. Any nursing unit that has no patient falls during a 30-day period is rewarded with a cookie party; units with no patient falls during a 60-day period are rewarded with a pizza party. The Weekly Falls Review Team was recognized by ANA at the Fourth Annual NDNQI Data Use Conference. The poster presented at this conference is on display during the Nurses Week Celebra-

NDNQI Case Studies in Nursing Quality Improvement

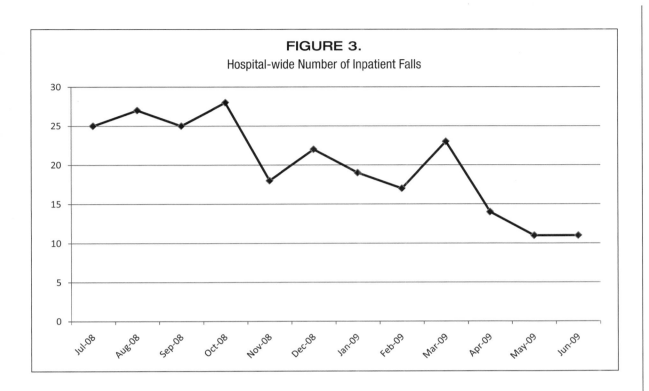

FIGURE 3.

Hospital-wide Number of Inpatient Falls

tion at CSM. Following the successful Weekly Falls Review Team model, the CSM Pressure Ulcer Team has recently implemented weekly review meetings. This team, including the direct-care nurse who identifies a pressure ulcer either at the time of admission or during the admission, meets weekly to review their pressure ulcer findings.

Conclusion

The most important part of the entire process was fostering individual nurse's accountability for patient safety and for implementation of prevention strategies. The Weekly Falls Review Team meetings, which examine *every* fall that occurs, transformed the nursing staff from accepting the belief that patients would fall to assuming accountability for preventing their patients from falling. Nurses want to provide safe care to each of their patients, not because a government agency or other regulatory body dictates it, but because it is the right thing to do. Providing safe patient care is the essence of nursing.

The Institute for Healthcare Improvement (2010) notes:

> *Although there is a considerable body of literature on falls prevention, little evidence exists for the absolute impact of any given intervention. Yet, we find that when health professionals believe that they can prevent falls in hospitals and undertake well-thought-out improvement programs, remarkable success can be achieved.*

Adopting an evidence-based fall prevention protocol and establishing an interprofessional Weekly Falls Review Team proved this at CHRISTUS St. Michael Health System. Nurses demonstrated their impact as patient advocates by leading the design and implementation of this quality improvement program. The program exemplifies an effective interprofessional approach that incorporates each discipline's unique view of patient falls so that barriers to fall prevention are quickly identified and remedied.

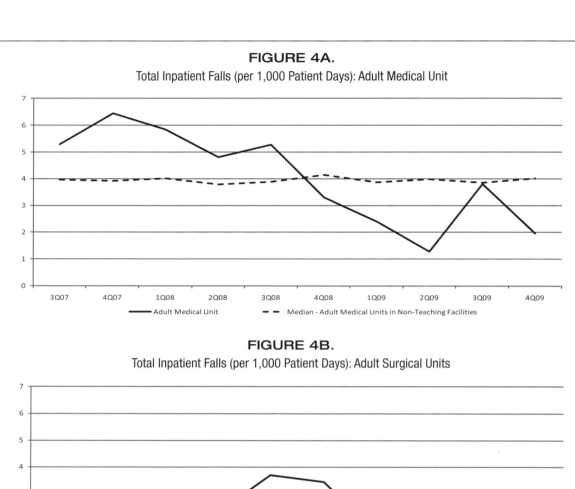

FIGURE 4A.

Total Inpatient Falls (per 1,000 Patient Days): Adult Medical Unit

——— Adult Medical Unit   – – – Median - Adult Medical Units in Non-Teaching Facilities

FIGURE 4B.

Total Inpatient Falls (per 1,000 Patient Days): Adult Surgical Units

——— Adult Surgical Units   – – – Median - Adult Surgical Units in Non-Teaching Facilities

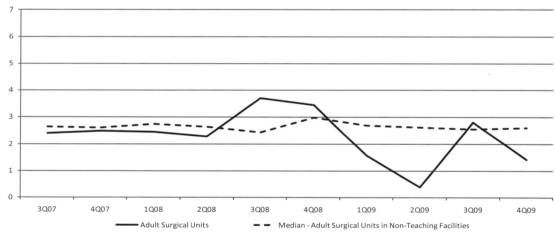

FIGURE 4C.

Total Inpatient Falls (per 1,000 Patient Days): Adult Medical-Surgical Units

——— Adult Medical/Surgical Combined Units   – – – Median - Adult Med-Surg Units in Non-Teaching Facilities

References

All URLs were retrieved on December 10, 2010.

Centers for Medicare & Medicaid Services (CMS). (2007). *Changes to the hospital inpatient prospective payment systems and fiscal year rates.* GAO-07-1200R. http://www.gao.gov/decisions/majrule/d071200r.htm

Geller, K. H., & Guzman, J. L. (2005). *Focus: JCAHO 2005 national patient safety goals.* http://www.fojp.com/Focus_2005_1.pdf

Institute for Healthcare Improvement (IHI). (2010). *Reducing harm from falls.* http://www.ihi.org/IHI/Topics/PatientSafety/ReducingHarmfromFalls

Institute of Medicine (IOM). (2000). *To err is human: Building a safer health system.* Washington, DC: National Academies Press.

Joint Commission. (2005). *National patient safety goals for hospitals.* http://www.jointcommission.org/patientsafety/nationalpatientsafetygoals/

Two-Tier Fall Precautions Combined with Improved Staffing and New Equipment Reduce Injury Fall Rates

Scott Madaris, MSHSA, BSN, RN
Director of Clinical Education/Nursing Quality/Magnet Program Director
Scott_Madaris@memorial.org

Memorial Hospital
Chattanooga, Tennessee
www.memorial.org

Case Study Highlights

A two-tier approach to fall prevention led to zero injury falls on six medical and surgical units. New bed alarms, an algorithm for sitter usage, and a lower nurse–patient ratio were key structural changes that helped sustain the improvement. Lessons learned from post-fall huddles will be used to continue injury fall prevention efforts.

Quality Measurement and Organizational Structure

In January 2005, Memorial Hospital (see Figure 1) chose to participate in NDNQI® as an opportunity to seek out national nursing quality benchmarks. As Memorial moved forward in utilizing nursing-sensitive data, a shared governance design was formulated to involve bedside nurses in practice decisions and nursing-related policies. Memorial's Nurse Practice Council membership has evolved over time and is now composed of an elected staff nurse chair and co-chair, voting members from all inpatient and outpatient nursing areas, and non-voting representatives from the Pharmacy, Advanced Practice Nursing, Quality, and Risk Management departments.

Over the last two years, the Nursing Quality Council was redesigned and incorporated with the Nurse Practice Council. This merger brought quality decisions that affect clinical practice to the forefront, empowering nursing staff to provide insight and be involved with quality improvement. With this change in governance structure there have been several initiatives, including fall reduction, that have brought more evidence-based practices to the bedside.

Problem Identification

The Restraint and Fall Committee examined monthly fall data and used NDNQI benchmarks to evaluate total and injury fall rates. In November 2007, discussion about revising the existing fall prevention program began. Staff and nursing leadership determined that the previous fall program was no longer effective. Multiple acute care nursing units had injury fall rates above the NDNQI mean in 3Q07 and there had been several falls with major injuries.

FIGURE 1.
Facility Profile

Memorial Hospital
Chattanooga, Tennessee
www.memorial.org

Facility overview	Memorial Hospital is a faith-based facility in the southeast region of the Tennessee Valley specializing in Orthopedic, Cardiac, and Oncology services. Memorial Hospital's mission is to nurture the healing ministry of the Church in the twenty-first century, emphasizing human dignity and social justice in the creation of healthier communities. Memorial Hospital has participated in NDNQI since January 2005.
Teaching status	Non-teaching
Ownership status	Not-for-profit
Magnet® status	Applying for Magnet recognition
Staffed beds	336
Affiliations	Catholic Health Initiatives
Awards	Leapfrog Top 50 Hospitals, 2006 Thomson Reuters 100 Top Cardiovascular Hospitals, 2006 (fourth time) Thomson Reuters 100 Top Hospitals (Overall), 2009 (sixth consecutive year and seventh overall) "Consumer's Choice" by National Research, 2007 (sixth time) One of Tennessee's Best Employers by Business TN magazine, 2008 (fourth time)

The Restraint and Fall Committee noted several factors contributing to injury falls. At this time, patients were assessed for fall risk using clinical judgment, not a risk assessment tool. Fall signage was either being ignored by staff or not placed appropriately based on clinical assessment. Falls were often associated with patients getting up to use the bathroom. The Committee began working to design a prevention program, with the goal of achieving a zero injury fall rate.

Development of a Two-Tier Fall Reduction Program

To improve fall risk assessment and fall signage, the Committee gathered information about current practice, policy, and clinical tools. Fall identification bracelets with a "falling star" were already being used to distinguish at-risk patients, but assessment of risk needed to be standardized. The literature spoke of signage that not only alerted staff to potential fall risk, but also involved the patients, family, and visitors. Thus, new risk assessment tools and "traffic light" signs were trialed on two units with high-risk populations and increased fall rates.

After the trial, nursing staff said that the new fall signage was helpful and prompted triggers related to fall criteria, room clutter, and the use of fall risk identification bracelets. However, they stated the assessment tools were cumbersome and that "most patients became fall risks" based on the criteria used. After further discussion and analysis, it was concluded that most patients in the healthcare setting are at risk for falls, which generated discussion of a two-tier fall prevention process.

The first tier utilizes the concept of "standard" fall precautions for all acute care patients and includes basic fall reduction techniques, such as patient and family education, reduction of room clutter, placing the patient call light in reach, use of slipper socks, and utilization of assistive devices such as gait belts with transfer and ambulation. The second tier applies to patients with advanced age, equipment (such as IV pumps or other attached equipment), history of falls within the past year, or physical or cognitive impairments. At the second tier, patients would be placed on "strict" fall precautions which initially included fall signage (alert bracelets, yellow socks, "traffic light" signs, and

NDNQI Case Studies in
Nursing Quality Improvement

so forth), and hourly rounding. Bed alarms were later added for second-tier patients. These fall precautions were designed to catch falls before they happened, thereby reducing the risk of injury.

Implementation of the Fall Reduction Program

After the Nurse Practice Council provided feedback regarding the two-tier program changes, the program was re-piloted with utilization of the "traffic light" (see Figure 2) to alert staff, patients, and families to second-tier patients. The program was rolled out via an electronic education module that included a program for clinical staff as well as a program for all staff (e.g., nutrition services, maintenance, and environmental service personnel). The program went live hospital-wide after education in March 2008. Fall reduction education was also incorporated in the annual Nursing Skills Day and the nursing orientation process.

Continued Structure and Process Changes to Prevent Falls

After realizing the scope and depth of the fall reduction project as well as a need for continued emphasis on fall prevention, the Restraint and Fall Committee was separated after the initiation of the two-tier program. The Fall Committee became a subcommittee of the Nurse Practice Council, allowing clinical staff to be more directly involved in evaluating effectiveness of the fall reduction program.

As part of the Nursing Practice Council, the Fall Committee initiated further improvements. With top-level leadership support, new beds were purchased in May 2008. The purchased beds incorporated alarms as an intervention for patients on strict fall precautions. As total falls per 1,000 patient days continued to be above the NDNQI median for some units in the first quarter of 2008, there was a review of how sitters were being used in the organization and a new algorithm was created for sitter usage in July 2008. In the same month, nursing leadership also initiated

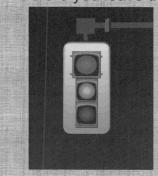

FIGURE 2.
Memorial Healthcare System "Traffic Light" Sign

Please Help to Decrease Falls at Memorial Healthcare System

Before you leave the patient's room, check:

- ✓ Is the patient's room free of clutter, spills, and other fall hazards?
- ✓ Is patient bed in lowest position, with brakes locked, and with 2 side rails up?
- ✓ Are Call Light/phone/personal items within reach?
- ✓ Is Fall Alert Armband on patient?
- ✓ Was bed alarm checked?

nurse–patient ratio changes on acute care units of one nurse to four to five patients during day shifts and one nurse to six patients during night shifts with the goal of nurses spending more time at the bedside to sustain improved clinical outcomes. (See Figure 3.)

In October through December 2008, a post-fall form was created. Reviewing post-fall data, the Fall Committee identified a trend in falls occurring two to three hours after patients over the age of 65 received sleep aids. Recommendations from the Nursing Practice Council and Medication Management Committee were made to restrict usage of sedatives for sleep. These restrictions were incorporated into physician standing orders.

During this same time, nursing leadership began to pilot several other initiatives, including the use of chair alarms. Several clinical areas were involved in these pilots, including medical telemetry (1 Central) and surgical telemetry (2 South) units. Chair alarms were connected to the nurse call light system which sent an immediate alert if the alarm was activated. As of result of the successful pilot test, chair alarms were placed on all inpatient nursing units in 2009.

FIGURE 3.
Unit Profiles

Overview This case study highlights improvements on six medical and/or surgical units, which serve a variety of adult patient populations.

			3Q07		3Q08	
Unit	Specialty	Staffed Beds	Total NHPPD	Hours Supplied by RNs (%)	Total NHPPD	Hours Supplied by RNs (%)
1 Central	Medical telemetry	34	10.49	62.4	10.92	61.6
1 North	Medical telemetry	24	8.71	63.4	9.98	66.2
1 South	Medical telemetry	24	8.66	56.6	11.05	62.3
2 South	Surgical telemetry	33	10.25	62.5	11.08	63.8
5 South	Surgical	30	9.19	68.3	10.92	68.1
4 South	Medical–surgical	28	8.37	66.6	10.19	66.8

Note: NHPPD = Nursing hours per patient day.

Also in 2009, the Fall Committee created standing orders for post-fall patient care. Post-fall huddles were implemented during which the patient's nurse, certified nursing assistant, charge nurse, and unit manager would immediately discuss questions related to type and severity of the fall, events leading up to the fall, staffing, and prevention measures. Lessons learned from the post-fall huddles will be used to further improve fall prevention practices.

Monitoring Progress and Celebrating Success

After the two-tier fall reduction program was implemented in March 2008, injury fall rates decreased substantially (see Figures 4A, 4B, and 4C). The additional structure and process changes implemented by the Nursing Practice Council helped maintain this success. Three units achieved zero injury falls for four consecutive quarters (1 North, 4 South, and 5 South). Two additional units had three quarters with no injuries (1 South and 2 South). To recognize their success, a

monthly trophy was awarded to those areas with noted improvements below the NDNQI benchmarks.

Ongoing Commitment to Fall Reduction

In 2Q09, most units' injury fall rates rose toward or above the NDNQI median, although generally not to previous levels. Memorial Hospital recognizes the continued challenges within the realm of fall reduction (multiple competing care priorities, fully integrating new staff, etc.). The hospital will continue working toward the goal of zero falls. Beginning in July 2010, several evidence-based practice initiatives from the hospital's parent organization, Catholic Health Initiatives, have been incorporated into the fall management program, including re-education of all staff and implementation of the Morse Fall Scale. Further restriction of sleep aids has also been recommended. The nursing staff and leadership at Memorial Hospital will continue to participate in NDNQI and strive to prevent falls and resulting injuries.

NDNQI Case Studies in Nursing Quality Improvement

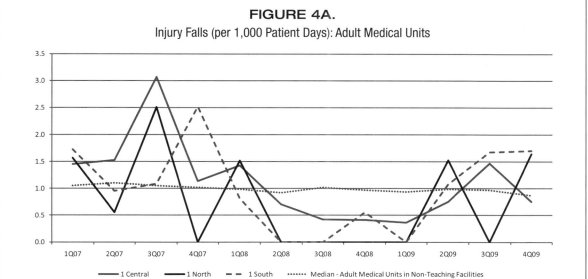

FIGURE 4A.

Injury Falls (per 1,000 Patient Days): Adult Medical Units

1 Central — 1 North — 1 South ······· Median - Adult Medical Units in Non-Teaching Facilities

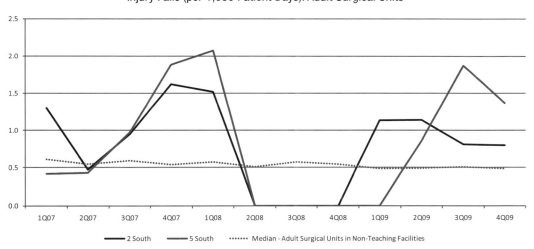

FIGURE 4B.

Injury Falls (per 1,000 Patient Days): Adult Surgical Units

2 South — 5 South ······· Median - Adult Surgical Units in Non-Teaching Facilities

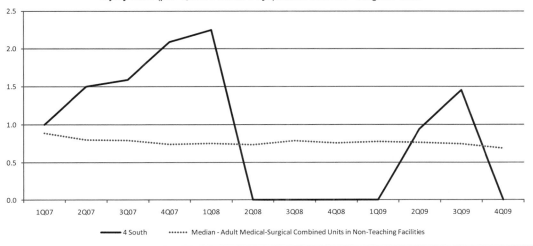

FIGURE 4C.

Injury Falls (per 1,000 Patient Days): Adult Medical–Surgical Units

4 South ······· Median - Adult Medical-Surgical Combined Units in Non-Teaching Facilities

Multiple Practice Changes Promote a Culture of Shared Responsibility to Reduce Patient Falls and Fall Injuries

Marilyn S. Mokracek, MSN, RN, CCRN, NE-BC
Nurse Manager
mmokracek@sleh.com

Cheryl Novak Lindy, PhD, RN-BC, NEA-BC
Director, Nursing and Patient Education and Research

St. Luke's Episcopal Hospital
Houston, Texas
www.stlukeshouston.com

Case Study Highlights

New equipment and additional staff were combined with safety huddles, visual cues communicating risk status, and immediate post-fall debriefing to reduce total and injury falls. These changes fostered a philosophy of shared responsibility for patient safety. After two years of success, injury fall rates began to trend upward and additional best practice interventions are being pursued.

Fall Rates above NDNQI Benchmark Spur Quality Improvement

In 2006, fall rates at St. Luke's Episcopal Hospital (see Figure 1) indicated an opportunity for improvement in preventing patient falls and fall injuries. On the medical and rehabilitation units, the eight-quarter averages for total falls per 1,000 patient days *were* higher than the corresponding NDNQI® eight-quarter average median. Injury fall rates for the same units were equal

to or below the eight-quarter NDNQI means. The hospital's Best Practice Council facilitated a multi-faceted fall prevention initiative that was combined with new equipment and additional staff time to successfully reduce falls and related injuries throughout the hospital.

Best Practice Council Creates Fall Prevention Team

St. Luke's Best Practice Council was created in September 2006 to replace the nursing quality program as a mechanism to promote performance improvement through evidence-based outcomes. The previous nursing quality program focused on nursing documentation compliance instead of performance improvement and patient outcomes. The Best Practice Council changed the focus to investigating patient outcomes variances and providing evidence-based direction for clinical change to enhance quality patient care. The Best Practice Council identifies quality problems

FIGURE 1.
Facility Profile

St. Luke's Episcopal Hospital
Houston, Texas
www.stlukeshouston.com

Facility overview	St. Luke's Episcopal Hospital is a large metropolitan teaching hospital in southeast Texas. St. Luke's provides general tertiary care on 9 critical care units and 17 step-down, medical, surgical, and rehabilitation units. St. Luke's has participated in NDNQI since 1999.
Teaching status	Academic medical center
Ownership status	Not-for-profit
Magnet® status	Magnet-designated since 2001
Staffed beds	553
Affiliations	Texas Medical Center
Awards	First hospital in Texas to achieve ANCC Magnet Designation

and creates interprofessional teams to review and test evidence-based practices. These smaller teams identify promising interventions and test them in the current environment to ensure positive impact. The team then makes recommendations to the larger Best Practice Council, which then mandates the practice change throughout the organization.

The Patient Falls Prevention Best Practice Team was one of the first teams created by the larger Council in September 2006. The team leader and membership were selected from multiple units and disciplines. Team members included nursing staff and manage-

ment, physical therapy, radiology, clinical nurse specialists, and nursing research. The team was directed to identify and implement best practices to reduce the number of patient falls. The team's original goal was to reduce total falls per 1,000 patient days to 2.0 or fewer, with no moderate or serious injury.

Development of the Falls Prevention Initiative

The team assessed the hospital's current practice and outcomes data. Retrospective chart review demon-

FIGURE 2.
Unit Profiles

Overview This case study highlights improvements on three nursing units serving a variety of adult patient populations.

Unit	Specialty	Staffed Beds	Total NHPPD	Hours Supplied by RNs (%)	RNs with BSN Degree (%)	RNs with National Certification (%)	Average RN Experience (years)
17 Tower	Rehabilitation	24	7.05	62.9	28	57	12.3
20 Tower	Oncology	34	7.33	63.6	62	0	7.3
21 Tower	Medical	34	7.32	63.4	38	19	8.3

Note: NHPPD = Nursing hours per patient day.

NDNQI Case Studies in
Nursing Quality Improvement

strated patients were correctly assessed and identified as being at risk for falls, but interventions to prevent falls were not consistently implemented or documented by nursing staff. After evaluating current practice, the team reviewed recent research (Krauss, Evanoff, Hitcho, Ngugi, Dunagan et al., 2005; Mills, Neily, Luan, Stalhandske, & Weeks, 2005). The review of falls prevention literature revealed three recommendations for practice change:

• Visual cues that communicate risk level,

• Safety huddles at the start of each shift, and

• Immediate debriefing following a fall.

Beginning January 2007, the team decided to pilot the recommendations on select acute care units (see Figure 2) representing a variety of specialties, including the medical, oncology, and rehabilitation units.

Visual cues quickly alert all hospital staff that a patient is at risk of falling. Yellow-colored non-skid socks were selected to identify patients at risk of falling. In addition, a yellow sign was posted on patients' room doors and on the front of their charts. If patients had previously fallen, they received red socks. Hospital staff were educated to ensure that anyone seeing a patient in the hall with red socks knew the patient should always be accompanied and not left alone. Visual reminders were posted in patients' rooms and bathrooms, including safety signage (see Figure 3) and a stop sign.

Second, the Patient Falls Prevention Best Practice Team developed a safety huddle (see Figure 4). The unit staff implemented the huddle as part of change-of-shift discussion on each patient care unit. During the safety huddle, patients at a high risk for falls were identified and labeled "community property" and every staff member took responsibility for the patient's safety. All staff responds to a patient's call light regardless of the patient's RN assignment. During the pilot phase, the team ascertained that staff acceptance and participation in the program directly correlated with the degree of the nurse manager's commitment and participation. Therefore, each unit nurse manager was

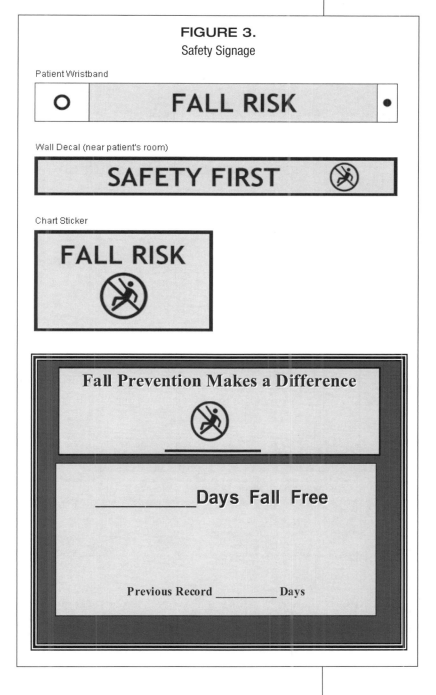

FIGURE 3.
Safety Signage

directed by the Best Practice Council to personally lead the unit huddle.

Third, a fall reporting and debriefing procedure was adopted to detail specific responses following a fall, including a debriefing with the nursing supervisor within one hour of every fall. Timely reporting of

FIGURE 4.
Shift Huddle Form

"HUDDLE"@ SHIFT START

DATE: _____ TIME _____

High Fall Risk Patients

Room	Name	Toileting Sched.	Bed Alarm	PCC

Completed Form in Binder/Notebook Before Shift End
PS-5921 01/2009   *Not A Part of the Permanent Medical Record*

"HUDDLE"@ SHIFT START

"PREVENT A FALL" ACTIONS

- 2 Hour toileting schedule ☺
  - *Even Rooms on Even Hours –*
  - *Odd Rooms on Odd Hours*
  - *"It's Time to Assist You to the BR or BSC"*
- OOB in chair for meals
- Bed Alarm "Rings" and US will page to "all staff"
  - *Staff Closest to Room Will Respond*
- Prompt Response to Call Light by All Staff
  - *Patient is Community Property: The Patient Belongs to Everyone*
- **RN determines off unit transportation mode**
- **Never** leave a patient alone in the bathroom or on BSC
- Socks:
  - **Yellow = High Fall Risk   Red = Patient has Fallen**

Resource: AM _____ PM _____

Note: PCC = After meals; BR = Bathroom; BSC = Bedside commode; OOB = Out of bed; US = Unit secretary.

---

critical information coupled with prompt staff feedback regarding the event created a heightened awareness and focus on prevention of patient falls. To mitigate any fall-related injuries, the Patient Falls Prevention Best Practice Team decided to utilize the expertise of the hospital's Rapid Response Team, which consists of a critical care RN, a respiratory therapist, and a medical resident. The critical care RN conducts an advance assessment to determine injury. If any noticeable injury or head trauma occurred during the fall, the critical care RN follows up at specific intervals to reassess and identify any further complications. The medical resident writes orders and conducts tests and procedures as needed. The Rapid Response Team may be activated by any RN concerned about changes in a patient's condition. However, immediate notification and activation of the Rapid Response Team is now mandatory for all patient falls.

New Equipment, Additional Staff, and Accountability Support Fall Prevention

Nursing administration's support proved critical to the success of the plan. In support of the initiative, financial

NDNQI Case Studies in Nursing Quality Improvement

resources were dedicated to fall prevention. Bed and chair exit alarms were purchased during the pilot phase for every patient room in 2007. At the same time, a new patient call system was installed, which alerted the entire unit when a bed exit alarm was activated.

A Patient Care Companion role was created to act as unit-specific "sitters". With the 2008 nursing budget, 22.2 additional full-time employees (FTEs) were assigned to units with high fall-risk populations. Nursing administration also created a unit-based Safety Coach role to educate staff and monitor compliance with safety initiatives. Safety coaches receive quarterly training in the latest initiatives designed to prevent patient falls. Eight hours of administrative time are dedicated to enable the safety coaches to attend the training each quarter. The unit-specific safety coaches act as a role model and mentor for peers regarding patient safety issues.

Nursing leaders were committed to the belief that all employees are responsible for ensuring patient safety and fall prevention. Therefore, patient safety was added as a performance standard on all employees' annual performance appraisals. Employees are held accountable for patient safety, including fall prevention in performance of their daily patient care work activities.

Each unit's compliance with the preventing falls initiatives was reported to all unit managers and directors monthly. The unit staff and management team were charged with developing individualized action plans to increase compliance on deficient units. Compliance with the shift huddle was monitored quarterly by the chair of the Patient Falls Prevention Best Practice Team by random sampling of unit huddle forms. These results were tracked and reported to nurse managers and directors.

Educating Staff about Best Practices for Fall Prevention

Mandatory fall prevention training was offered on all shifts so that staff could easily attend. All nurse manag-

ers, assistant nurse managers, and supervisors received training specifically aimed at conducting the post-fall debriefing. Emphasis was placed on variances that led to the fall and coaching staff on interventions to prevent future patient falls. The Medical–Surgical Education Specialist rounded on each unit and attended unit staff meetings to conduct staff education needs assessments. The Education Specialist also conducted fall event management quality monitoring after each patient fall. Additional staff training was provided as needed.

Monitoring Patient Falls Data

Patient falls are reported electronically with an online occurrence reporting form. Once completed by the RN assigned to the patient, this is automatically routed to the unit nurse manager for immediate review and investigation. Monthly reports for unit-specific patient falls and patient falls with injury are posted online and accessible to all hospital management. Managers use these internal monthly reports to identify trends for early intervention. Data also are extracted from the occurrence reporting form and uploaded to NDNQI quarterly for national benchmarking.

Outcomes data demonstrated a progressive decrease in total and injury falls on the pilot units, so the plan was subsequently implemented throughout the hospital. Implementing these best practices resulted in fewer falls and fall injuries. (See Figures 5A and 5B.) In particular, the medical and rehabilitation units had numerous quarters with injury fall rates below the NDNQI median.

The success of the plan continues to be evaluated using outcomes data. Average total and injury fall rates remain below the NDNQI median for medical and rehabilitation units. However, several units had higher fall rates in the fourth quarter of 2009. Therefore, the team is currently investigating interventions to prevent falls in patients demonstrating impulsive behavior. Additionally, the Patient Falls Prevention Best Practice Team conducted another review of the literature and is currently piloting hourly rounding on all high-

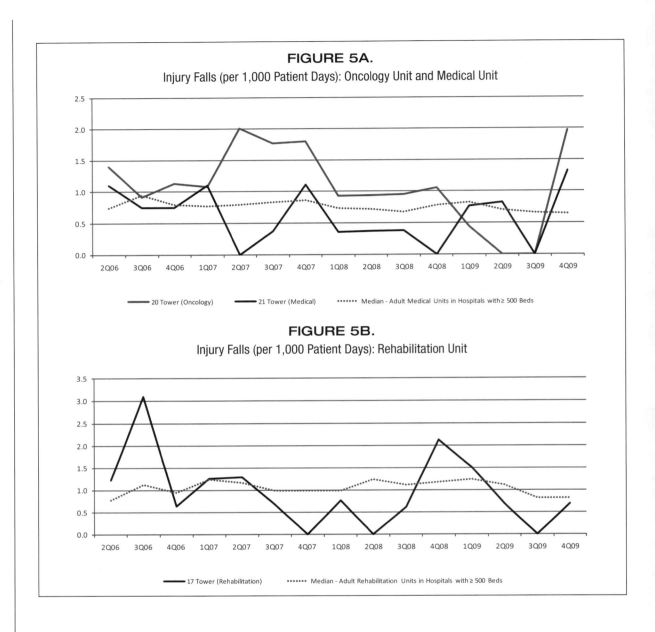

FIGURE 5A.

Injury Falls (per 1,000 Patient Days): Oncology Unit and Medical Unit

——— 20 Tower (Oncology)   ——— 21 Tower (Medical)   ••••••• Median - Adult Medical Units in Hospitals with ≥ 500 Beds

FIGURE 5B.

Injury Falls (per 1,000 Patient Days): Rehabilitation Unit

——— 17 Tower (Rehabilitation)   ••••••• Median - Adult Rehabilitation Units in Hospitals with ≥ 500 Beds

risk patients focusing on the 5 Ps: Pain, Potty, Pantry, Position, and Patient Environment.

References

Krauss, M., Evanoff, B., Hitcho, E., Ngugi, K., Dunagan, W., Fischer, I., Birge, S., Johnson, S., Costantinou, E., &

Fraser, V. (2005). A case-control study of patient-, medication-, and care-related risk factors for inpatient falls. *Journal of General Internal Medicine, 20*(2), 116–122.

Mills, P., Neily, J., Luan, D., Stalhandske, E., & Weeks, W. (2005). Using aggregate root cause analysis to reduce falls and related injuries. *Joint Commission Journal on Quality and Patient Safety, 31*(1), 21–31.

Reducing Catheter-Associated Urinary Tract Infections in the Surgical Intensive Care Unit

Barbara Ochsner, MS, RN
RN/Clinical Director, Resource Services
bjo1@pvhs.org

Medical Center of the Rockies
Loveland, Colorado
www.pvhs.org

Case Study Highlights

Staff nurses on the quality improvement team worked to eliminate catheter-associated urinary tract infections (CAUTIs) by adding a review of the necessity of a urinary catheter to the daily interprofessional rounds. Primary infection prevention was found to be far more cost-effective than present-on-admission screening.

Identification of the CAUTI Problem

In early 2008, advanced practice nurses and quality improvement staff at the Medical Center of the Rockies (MCR; see Figure 1) recognized that the CAUTI rate on the Surgical Intensive Care Unit (SICU; see Figure 2) was above the NDNQI® mean in the fourth quarter of 2007. This continued for the first two quarters of 2008. When the problem with CAUTI rates was identified, the organization's process improvement methodology, the Plan-Do-Check-Act (PDCA) cycle, was activated. A PDCA team was formed consisting of staff RNs, a clinical nurse specialist (CNS), an infection prevention and control RN, the patient safety officer, an education nurse specialist, and a wound/ostomy nurse. Building on the existing quality monitoring program, the PDCA team investigated the specific

causes of CAUTIs on the SICU, and then implemented evidence-based practice (EBP) changes that eliminated CAUTIs for 5 consecutive quarters.

Quality Monitoring on the SICU

RNs in the SICU are well informed about the quality of care they are providing. The nurse manager and CNS provide regular updates on patient outcomes through verbal communication and by posting NDNQI results on the unit for review. SICU staff nurses are active on both the Critical Care Standards of Care Committee (SOC) and the organizational Nursing Quality Committee. Nursing-sensitive indicators, including CAUTIs, are reviewed regularly at these committee meetings. When CAUTI rates increased above the NDNQI mean, the PDCA team began the Planning phase, setting goals and initiating in-depth review of each CAUTI case to identify contributing factors.

Development of the Quality Improvement Initiative

The PDCA team set the following goals: review 2007 CAUTI data at MCR, identify EBP processes for

FIGURE 1.
Facility Profile

Medical Center of the Rockies (MCR)
Loveland, Colorado
www.pvhs.org

Facility overview	Opened in February 2007, MCR is a tertiary-care community hospital in northern Colorado. The facility is a Level II trauma center with 24 intensive care beds (12 surgical/trauma, 12 cardiac). MCR has participated in NDNQI since 2007.
Teaching status	Non-teaching
Ownership status	Private, not-for-profit
Magnet® status	Application submitted in February 2010
Staffed beds	112
Affiliations	Poudre Valley Health System (PVHS)
Awards	Malcolm Baldrige National Quality Award, 2008

urinary catheter care, identify areas for implementation of improvements, and provide recommendations for improvement to the EBP committee (a subcommittee of the Nursing Quality Committee). The team defined its success measure as a 75%–100% reduction of CAUTI rates by July 2008.

As the PDCA team investigated the 2007 CAUTI cases, it found the average age of the patient who developed a CAUTI was 73.3 years. The incidents were evenly split between males and females and the average time to infection for a patient in the SICU was approximately 4.5 days. Notably, patients who developed a CAUTI were most often those who were assessed to be a high fall risk. The team hypothesized that some of the infections were related to the prolonged use of the catheter to decrease the patient's movement to the bathroom in an effort to reduce the likelihood of a fall.

Evidence-based practice recommendations stated that removal of the urinary catheter as early as possible is very effective in CAUTI prevention (Smith, 2003; Senese, Hendricks, Morrison, & Harris, 2005). Silver-coated catheters were also noted as an effective prevention measure (Rupp et al., 2005). No special perineal care techniques were recommended in the EBP literature. The perineal area should be cleaned with soap and water prior to sterile insertion of the

FIGURE 2.
Unit Profile

Overview The Surgical Intensive Care Unit (SICU) serves adult patients with trauma and medical–surgical critical care needs. The SICU received the AACN Beacon Award for Excellence in 2008.

Unit	Staffed Beds	Total NHPPD	Hours Supplied by RNs (%)	RNs with BSN Degree (%)	RNs with National Certification (%)	Average RN Experience (years)
SICU	12	19.7	92	65	55	12

Note: NHPPD = Nursing hours per patient day.

NDNQI Case Studies in
Nursing Quality Improvement

catheter (Wong & Hooton, 1981; Gray, 2004). Antimicrobial solutions are not necessary and only routine hygiene is required for patients who have a urinary catheter in place (Gray, 2004; Newman, 2007). Therefore, the PDCA team determined the primary change needed was to standardize ongoing review of whether the patient still needed a urinary catheter or it could be discontinued. The team also initiated use of silver-coated catheters in March 2008.

Cost Analysis: Present on Admission Screening

As part of the EBP review, the PDCA team examined the costs and benefits of implementing urinary analysis at the time of catheter insertion to screen for infections that were present on admission. For each CAUTI not present on admission, there would be a potential payment reduction by the Centers for Medicare and Medicaid Services (CMS) of $676 per patient. Since there were 15 cases of CAUTI in the intensive care units (ICUs) in 2007, annual payments would have been reduced by $10,140. The lowest cost of a urinalysis (U/A) microtest was $16 and in 2007 there were approximately 650 patients admitted to the ICU. If 75% of these patients had a urinary catheter inserted, the cost of present-on-admission screening would be $7,800, a difference from the $10,400 total of approximately $2,600. The team determined that testing all ICU patients was not recommended. However, the PDCA team did recommend improvement of the documentation of the presence of a urinary catheter upon admission to the facility; the documentation requirements, which were not identified in the policy prior to the CAUTI improvement initiative, were detailed in a policy revision.

Intervention Roll-Out

The PDCA team submitted their recommendation for daily review of catheter necessity with the goal of implementing culture changes that supported the best practice of removing urinary catheters within 3 days of

insertion. A revised policy was reviewed with the SOC and Nursing Quality Committees and approved by the Nursing Policy and Procedures Committee. Prior to the implementation of this practice change, the decision to remove a urinary catheter was based only on the patient's transfer to another unit providing a lower level of care or a reduction in the patient's fall risk. In the new process, review of catheter necessity was to be facilitated by the patient's assigned RN in collaboration with the patient's physician during interprofessional team rounds each day.

SICU staff nurses worked on designing posters to educate staff about why the change in practice was needed and how to measure the change. Training was focused on providing "world-class" patient care, with patient safety, comfort, and reduction of infection as the goal. Posters that explained the new procedure were displayed in places that would catch staff attention, such as the break room, the staff restrooms, and the report room. SICU RNs who were members of the Standards of Care Committee communicated the policy revisions and goals for CAUTI reduction to all nursing staff through emails, flyers, posters, and staff meetings. An incentive of a meal for staff (such as pizza for all shifts) was offered if the unit was able to decrease the incidence of CAUTI by 75% when the review of the results occurred in July.

Daily review of catheter use began in April and May of 2008. In the SICU, the rate of CAUTI was reduced to zero by the third quarter of 2008 and remained zero until the fourth quarter of 2009, when one severely compromised patient developed a CAUTI. (See Figure 3.) Most urinary catheters are now removed within 3 days of the patient's admission with the exception of patients with a clinical indication for the continuation of the catheter.

Celebrating Success

The implementation of best practices for urinary catheter use was extended to the remainder of the inpatient areas with similar success, although the SICU has

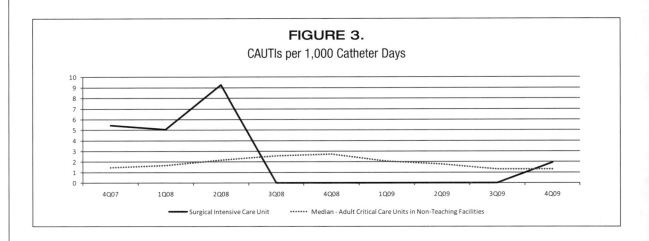

FIGURE 3.
CAUTIs per 1,000 Catheter Days

Surgical Intensive Care Unit .... Median - Adult Critical Care Units in Non-Teaching Facilities

been the most effective in achieving results quickly. Celebration of excellent clinical results included both individual RN and unit recognition for decreasing the number of infections through evidence-based process and policy changes. Accomplishments related to CAUTI rates were recognized in staff meetings, at the promised incentive meal, and in celebratory posters in the break room.

The PDCA team turned over ongoing monitoring of CAUTI rates and process improvements to the Infection Control Committee, which reports to the Nursing Quality Committee on a quarterly schedule. Initially, regular monitoring and feedback about daily catheter reviews supported the continued low infection rate on the SICU. As time progressed, staff nurses adopted the review of catheter necessity into their daily routines and the need to provide support decreased with the "hardwiring" of the changes. The nurses in the SICU have taken responsibility for assuring that their patients do not experience preventable complications during their stay. The nurse is present during the interprofessional team rounds and is responsible to provide feedback about whether the indwelling urinary catheter should be discontinued. The motivation of the staff nurses to bring about effective change for the patients was instrumental in the success of this initiative.

References

All URLs were retrieved December 10, 2010.

Gray, M. (2004). What nursing interventions reduce the risk of symptomatic urinary tract infection in the patient with an indwelling catheter? *Journal of Wound, Ostomy and Continence Nursing, 31*(1), 3–13.

Newman, D. (2007). The indwelling urinary catheter: Principles for best practice. *Journal of Wound, Ostomy and Continence Nursing, 34*(6), 655–661.

Rupp, M. E., Fitzgerald, T., Marion, N., Helget, V., Puumala, S., Anderson, J., & Fey, P. (2004). Effect of silver-coated urinary catheters: Efficacy, cost-effectiveness, and antimicrobial resistance. *American Journal of Infection Control, 32*(8), 445–449.

Senese, V., Hendricks, M. B., Morrison, M., & Harris, J. (2006). Clinical practice guidelines: Care of the patient with an indwelling catheter. *Urologic Nursing, 26*(1), 80–81. http://www.o-wm.com/content/internal-and-external-urinary-catheters-a-primer-clinical-practice

Smith, J. M. (2003). Indwelling catheter management: From habit-based to evidence-based practice. *Ostomy Wound Management, 49*(12), 34–45.

Wong, E. S., & Hooton, T. M. (1981). *Guidelines for prevention of catheter-associated urinary tract infections.* http://wonder.cdc.gov/wonder/prevguid/p0000416/p0000416.asp

Primary Line Insertion Team Reduced Central Line-Associated Blood Stream Infections in the Neonatal ICU

Tammy Hoff, MS, RN
NICU Nurse Manager
tammy.hoff@cookchildrens.org

Cook Children's Medical Center
Fort Worth, Texas
www.cookchildrens.org

Case Study Highlights

Two full-time nurses were hired as a dedicated, unit-based line insertion team. The team implemented evidence-based practices for line insertion and dressing changes. Daily rounds encouraging prompt removal of unused lines, combined with real-time feedback on infection-free days, further reduced infection rates. Root cause analysis of each infection provided learning opportunities for staff.

Identifying and Exploring the Problem of CLABSI

The Level IIIC Neonatal Intensive Care Unit (NICU) at Cook Children's Medical Center (CCMC) recognized that overall central line infections rates were above those in similar NICUs around the country. (See Figures 1 and 2 for profiles of CCMC, and its NICU, respectively.)

Monthly data on central line-associated blood stream infections (CLABSIs) were first collected according to National Healthcare Safety Network (NHSN) guide-lines. In 2006, the NICU's annual rate of infections per 1,000 central line days was 7.5, which was above the NHSN average of 5.8 infections per 1,000 central line days. In January 2007, the unit saw a spike in CLABSIs of 17 infections per 1,000 central line days.

When the unit looked at potential causes of the infections it became clear that there was no consistency in how any of the central lines were managed. Over 50 physicians and neonatal nurse practitioners were able to place peripherally inserted central catheters (PICC). Variations in central line insertion and maintenance practices were potentially contributing to the high infection rate. NICU leaders and staff began focusing on ways to decrease CLABSIs, especially by creating consistency in the processes associated with PICC lines.

Development of QI Initiative and Goals

A staff member who was a student in a nursing master's program suggested the idea of a PICC team to limit the number of clinicians who place those lines. This evidence-based suggestion was refined into a quality improvement (QI) plan centered on creating

Cook Children's Medical Center
Fort Worth, Texas
www.cookchildrens.org

Facility overview	Cook Children's Medical Center (CCMC) is a freestanding children's hospital in north central Texas. CCMC provides comprehensive tertiary care, including neonatal and pediatric intensive care, nephrology, neurology, oncology, surgery, cardiology, and much more. A large expansion project is scheduled to open in the spring of 2011. CCMC accommodates many education rotations but is not considered a teaching facility. CCMC has participated in NDNQI since October 2007.
Teaching status	Non-teaching
Ownership status	Not-for-profit
Magnet® status	Magnet-designated in 2006
Staffed beds	282
Affiliations	None
Awards	Ranked among America's best children's hospitals by *U.S. News & World Report*, 2009–2010 Top 100 Integrated Health Care Networks by SDI Health LLC, 2009–2010 Ranked 23rd on *The Dallas Morning News* list of top places to work

a two-person team to place and manage the majority of central lines on the unit. The hypothesis was that fewer people inserting and maintaining lines would create less of a chance for lapses from best practice techniques, ultimately decreasing CLABSIs and the substantial morbidity and mortality associated with these infections. The goal of achieving a 50% decrease in CLABSIs within the first 18 months of implementation was set.

Administrative Support and Cost-Benefit Analysis

A proposal for a dedicated unit-based line insertion team consisting of two full-time nurses was presented and accepted by hospital administration. This proposal coincided with a decrease in patient census in the NICU, which provided the opportunity to modify two existing nursing positions to PICC nurses without

FIGURE 2.
Unit Profile

Overview The Level IIIC Neonatal Intensive Care Unit (NICU) provides quaternary care, including extracorporeal membranous oxygenation (ECMO), hypothermia therapy, and high-frequency ventilation. Average daily census is 57. The NICU is recognized as a Center of Excellence by the Extracorporeal Life Support Organization.

Unit	Staffed Beds	Total NHPPD	Hours Supplied by RNs (%)	RNs with BSN Degree (%)	RNs with National Certification (%)	Average RN Experience (years)
NICU	76	15.4	98	78	30	7

Note: NHPPD = Nursing hours per patient day.

affecting the staffing level on the unit. The project was implemented with no additional full-time employees (FTEs) required and therefore incurred minimal initial costs. One of the nurses hired had experience in placing PICC lines and was able to train the other team member. Training took place over a one-month period. During this time both team members completed competency assessments on the insertion of PICC lines with the medical staff of the NICU. Since each case of CLABSI adds an estimated $34,508 to the cost of care, the PICC team proposal was highly cost-effective (O'Grady et al., 2002).

Implementation of the PICC Team and Infection Prevention Practices

The PICC team was established in July 2007. Once the two PICC nurses were hired and trained, a central line insertion and maintenance protocol was developed by the PICC team members, NICU leadership, Infection Control, and Neonatology. Using evidence from the literature in conjunction with guidelines from the CDC (Centers for Disease Control and Prevention), a protocol was developed for insertion and dressing change procedures based on techniques that had been shown to lower infection risk (Brooker & Keenan, 2007; Danks, 2006; Eggimann & Pittet, 2002; O'Grady et al., 2002; Rickard, 2003).

Once the PICC team and the new protocol were in place, NICU nursing staff were educated in a skills-week session as well as through email communications about the changes in insertion and line maintenance practices. In addition to this initial education, there has been ongoing education related to CLABSI prevention. The PICC team evaluates staff compliance with established protocols and reinforces critical behaviors within the unit.

The PICC team gained immediate support and buy-in from all parties, particularly because it was composed of one experienced nurse from the NICU and one externally-hired nurse with extensive neonatal nursing and PICC knowledge. It was evident that the exter-

nal member was extremely qualified and capable of developing the PICC project. Because of the PICC team's comfort level with the unit, NICU staff nurses felt confident following the guidelines they developed. The PICC team would also routinely assist with procedures so that they would remain proficient in other clinical skills, which helped sustain support for the PICC team by NICU staff.

The PICC team and new protocol were implemented as a fluid project, which allowed for flexibility in adding new procedures along the way. From 2007 to 2009, numerous changes regarding central line insertion and maintenance took place, which are summarized below.

July 2007

PICC team formed, protocol developed, and training began

August – December 2007

- PICC team responsible for all line insertions, dressing changes, line removals, and infection monitoring

- Comprehensive insertion checklist implemented, including full-barrier precautions and use of Chlora-Prep

- Daily evaluation of all central venous line dressings

- PRN (as needed) dressing changes using Chlora-Prep and Biopatch

February 2008

- Daily rounds focused on removal of inactive lines, with moderate physician and nursing buy-in achieved

- Standardized times set for mechanical valve hub changes

June 2008

- Root cause analysis conducted by PICC team for each infection, with email feedback to staff as an opportunity to learn from each infection

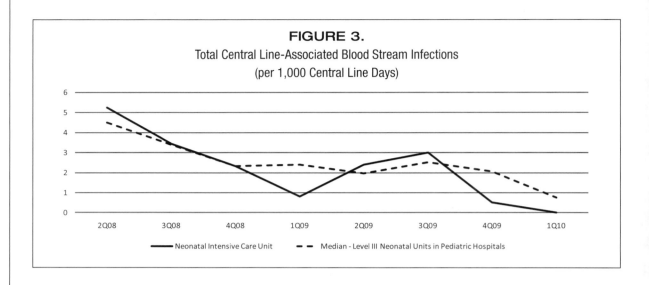

FIGURE 3.
Total Central Line-Associated Blood Stream Infections
(per 1,000 Central Line Days)

Neonatal Intensive Care Unit — — Median - Level III Neonatal Units in Pediatric Hospitals

- Current infection rate and number of infection-free days communicated to staff

- One-page physician order sheet developed to address pain management during insertion of PICC lines

January 2009

- Electronic sign installed in nursing lounges to provide real-time feedback on infection-free days

- Excellent physician and nursing support achieved for prompt removal of inactive heparin-locked central lines (considered for removal when not used for 24 hours)

- Family involvement with CLABSI reduction strategies (for instance, upon consent for a PICC line, families receive a one-page education sheet that encourages them to stop any staff member from touching their child if they have not seen the staff member engage in hand hygiene)

Monitoring Progress

Throughout this QI project, infection rates in the NICU were monitored by both the PICC team and the hospital infection control committee. The PICC team assessed each patient with a central line daily for signs and symptoms of infection. Blood cultures

were used to identify infections according to NHSN and NDNQI criteria. When the unit started reporting CLABSI rates to NDNQI in 2Q08, the total number of infections per 1,000 central line days had already decreased to 5.2. With growing acceptance of prompt line removal and the addition of root causes analysis for each infection, total CLABSI rates further declined to 0.8 in 1Q09. Annual infection rates decreased by 80%, from an average of 7.5 infections per 1,000 central line days in 2006 to an average of 1.7 in 2009 (see Figure 3).

In the second and third quarters of 2009, CLABSI rates rose slightly, although not to prior levels. Data were reviewed extensively for trends or any information that could explain the infections. No changes or lapses in practice were found. One positive blood culture that contributed to the infection rates during this time was determined to be a contaminant, as the infant had yeast growing on the skin but had no clinical signs of fungemia. Based on the longer trend line from 2006 to 2009, total CLABSI rates in mid-2009 were in line with the overall downward trend. In late 2009 and early 2010, infection rates continued to approach the zero mark, which is the unit's ultimate goal.

From the time that the PICC team was developed until achieving substantial results was approximately an 18-month period. During this time NICU leaders and staff adjusted procedures and learned many things that will help to keep infection rates as low as possible. Having a team dedicated to the topic of infections has been the biggest contribution to success. Implementing changes over an extended period has allowed the unit to incorporate new practices rather than being overwhelmed by numerous changes at one time. This has promoted a transformation in culture regarding central line infections. The NICU has been able to make CLABSI prevention part of the unit culture rather than just another QI project. Since combating CLABSIs is a never-ending process, the unit will continue to strive for the only acceptable rate: zero.

Celebration of Success

The current number of infection-free days is electronically displayed for staff members to see as they enter each lounge. When the unit reached 100 days infection-free, each staff member received a candy bar with a homemade wrapper that stated "Hooray 100 days infection free". When the unit reached 200 days, the hospital patient safety officer supplied the staff with a pizza party to celebrate that success.

The NICU has had so much success that other units in the hospital, as well as other neonatal ICUs around the area, have requested information on the NICU's practices, which it openly and willingly shares. The unit's successful reduction of CLABSIs was presented at a national nursing conference. The PICC team has traveled to evaluate other hospitals and give feedback on their current practice and suggestions for how to improve. NICU leaders and staff will keep working to maintain the success, share the story, and learn from others as the journey continues.

References

All URLs were retrieved on December 10, 2010.

Brooker, R. W., & Keenan, W. J. (2007). Catheter-related bloodstream infection following PICC removal in preterm infants. *Journal of Perinatology, 27*(3), 171–174.

Danks, L. A. (2006). Central venous catheters: A review of skin cleansing and dressings. *British Journal of Nursing, 15*(12), 650–654.

Eggimann, P., & Pittet, D. (2002). Overview of catheter-related infections with special emphasis on prevention based on educational programs. *Clinical Microbiology and Infection, 8*(5), 295–309.

O'Grady, N. P., Alexander, M., Dellinger, E. P., Gerberding, J. L., Heard, S. O., Maki, D. G. et al. (2002). Guidelines for the prevention of intravascular catheter-related infections. *Pediatrics, 110*(5), e51. http://pediatrics.aappublications.org/cgi/reprint/110/5/e51?maxtoshow=&hits=10&RESULTFORMAT=&fulltext=catheter&searchid=1&FIRSTINDEX=0&volume=110&issue=5&resourcetype=HWCIT

Rickard, N. (2003). Reducing infections associated with central venous catheters. *British Journal of Nursing, 12*(5), 274–282.

Pain Resource Nurse Program and Monthly Chart Audits Improve Pediatric Pain Assessment

Sonja Jones, MSN, RN, CPN
Nurse Manager, 4East/4South
joness@email.chop.edu

Renee Green, BSN, RN
Clinical Level III Staff Nurse, 4East/4South

Elizabeth Carroll, BSN, RN
Clinical Level III Staff Nurse, 4East/4South

Denise Zubczynski, BSN, RN, CPN
Clinical Level III Staff Nurse, 7West

Colleen Foster, BSN, RN
Clinical Level IV Staff Nurse, 7West

Susan M. Kolb, MSN, CRNP
Director, Advanced Practice Nursing

Beth Ely, PhD, RN
Nurse Researcher

Children's Hospital of Philadelphia
Philadelphia, Pennsylvania
www.chop.edu

Case Study Highlights

A combination of hospital-wide efforts and unique unit-based strategies led to improved pain assessment practices. Hospital-wide efforts included the development of a pain resource nurse (PRN) program with unit-based champions. Modification of the Patient Care Flowsheet was instrumental in improving pain assessment documentation. Unit-specific efforts included chart audits with direct individual coaching of nurses at the point of care.

FIGURE 1.
Facility Profile

Children's Hospital of Philadelphia (CHOP)
Philadelphia, Pennsylvania
www.chop.edu

Facility overview	The Children's Hospital of Philadelphia was the first pediatric hospital in the United States. Its physicians, nurses, researchers, and other professionals are recognized regionally and nationally for their expertise. CHOP's exceptional patient care and major research initiatives benefit children worldwide. CHOP has participated in NDNQI since 2004.
Teaching status	Academic medical center
Ownership status	Non-profit
Magnet® status	Magnet-designated since 2004
Staffed beds	443
Affiliations	None; freestanding facility with an ambulatory care network
Awards	Ranked as #1 pediatric hospital by *Parents* magazine
One of eight hospitals on *U.S. News & World Report* Honor Roll, 2010

Identification of the Problem

The Quality Practice and Patient Safety (QPPS) Council at Children's Hospital of Philadelphia (CHOP; see Figure 1) determined that its pain assessment-intervention-reassessment (AIR) cycle documentation was falling below the national median reported by NDNQI®. The need for improved pain management practices was reinforced when feedback from a Joint Commission visit in early 2007 indicated documentation of pain reassessment was inconsistent. Hospital-wide and unit-specific efforts from 2007 to 2009 have brought improvements in both frequency of pain assessments and the completion of AIR cycles.

Pain Resource Nurse Program

In the fall of 2006, CHOP hired several doctorally prepared nurses to form a center for nursing research and evidence-based practice. One of these nurses started a pain resource nurse program, bringing together nurses with an interest and expertise in pain management from all areas of practice represented in the hospital's QPPS Council. The group began meeting in December 2006 to identify areas of pain management that needed improvement and to promote a rapid turn-around time when planning and implementing any proposed changes. When the Joint Commission visit in early 2007 brought pain reassessment documentation to the forefront, nursing leadership identified the QPPS Council and the PRN subcommittee as the logical place to formulate and carry out an improvement plan. Nurses on the PRN subcommittee polled staff on their units and reviewed NDNQI data from the previous four quarters to better understand where and how to focus the improvement strategies.

Development of Hospital-Wide Initiatives

Three hospital-wide initiatives have improved pain management practices: revisions to the daily nursing documentation form, selection of a new assessment tool for children with cognitive impairment, and expansion of the PRN group's activities.

As of early 2007, charting pain management required access to three separate areas of the Patient Care Flowsheet as well as electronic charting of medication administration. On the front of the Patient Care Flowsheet, a pain intensity score was documented along with vital signs and daily weights. However, the interventions provided and subsequent pain reassessments were charted in a different section of the flowsheet. Finally, nursing notes related to pain were located at the back of the document. Nurses polled by the PRN group indicated that paper documentation was a major barrier to actually recording assessment scores since disjointed and duplicate documentation was required and they were often too busy.

Revisions to the daily nursing documentation form were made to co-locate all pain assessment data for a more logical flow of information. In addition, coded lists of common pain management interventions were provided, rather than having to repeatedly write out common interventions. The form was revised with input from QPPS, shared governance council members, and unit staff. In August 2007, the new flowsheet (see Figure 2) was rolled out with education at the hospital's QPPS Council meeting and through unit-level QPPS meetings.

The PRN subcommittee recognized the need to review evidence related to pain assessment in children with cognitive or neurologic impairment, a popula-

tion cared for frequently at this hospital. A small workgroup (staff nurses, clinical nurse specialists [CNSs], nurse researcher) was charged with this task. From an extensive literature review, the workgroup identified two promising pain assessment tools for children with cognitive impairment: the Pediatric Pain Profile (PPP) and the revised Face-Legs-Activity-Cry-Consolability (rFLACC) Scale (Hunt et al., 2004; Hunt et al., 2007; Malviya, Voepel-Lewis, Burke, Merkel, & Tait, 2006; Voepel-Lewis, Malviya, & Tait, 2005; Voepel-Lewis, Merkel, Tait, Trzcinka, & Malviya, 2002). The choice of these tools was based on their published psychometric properties as well as judgments about clinical utility by group members. Each tool was designed to include parents' input by identifying common pain behaviors of the child. To obtain feedback on applicability, clinical utility, preference for use, and time to complete for each tool, the tools were introduced to parents at the hospital's Family Advisory Council and to staff nurses through a formal quality improvement (QI) project.

Staff nurses on surgical (4East/4South) and rehabilitation units were asked to identify children with cognitive impairment and use the tools during every

---

FIGURE 2.
Revised Pain Management Documentation Flowsheet

Scale Legend

F=FLACC   WB=Wong-Baker FACES

N=Numeric   # = Nursing judgment

Pain Intervention Codes

0=Medication-Opioid	4=Music
1=Medication-Nonopioid	5=Repositioning
2=Distraction	6=Environmental modification
3=Relaxation	7=Other

P	Time																			
A	Scale Used																			
I	Pain Score																			
N	Interventions																			

Note: FLACC = Face–legs–activity–cry–consolability.

pain assessment (alternating the order of the tool each time they were used). The clinical units were chosen to capture both acute postoperative pain and more episodic pain. Bedside nurses and parents of children with cognitive impairment on these units completed a questionnaire about the tools. Through this process, the rFLACC tool was chosen and added to the CHOP pain management policy. To implement the tool, education was completed through QPPS, the PRN subcommittee, nursing grand rounds, posters, and individual discussion during the follow-up unit auditing process.

Through 2007–2009, the PRN subcommittee sustained and expanded its work. At PRN meetings, clinical pain management challenges are discussed and relevant articles from the literature are reviewed to provide ideas for enhancing practice. PRN members share successful education strategies and brainstorm about how to effect positive change in pain management practice. Child life specialists, psychologists, and pain nurse practitioners have joined the PRN group to expand its scope and provide interprofessional perspectives. Updates are received from workgroups tackling specific problems and are reported monthly to QPPS so the communication loop is complete. At the start of each QPPS Council meeting, unit representatives discuss their specific activities so other units can use or adapt their successes or help brainstorm solutions together. This ongoing conversation has proved to be invaluable in promoting communication within such a complex organization. Two units' pain assessment improvement stories are highlighted here.

Unit-Specific Improvement Initiatives: 4East/4South

Problem Identification

Pain management has always been a priority on the pediatric surgical/trauma unit, as each patient has the potential for significant pain related to treatment and recovery. While the institution was beginning to look at pain reassessment documentation, the 4East/4South (see Figure 3) leadership recognized that unit practices needed to be reviewed as well, without necessarily waiting for the centralized system to provide feedback. The unit's Patient Satisfaction Survey results were reviewed, paying special attention to the results relevant to pain management.

Development of QI Initiative and Goals

The unit's initial step was to revise the electronic Medication Administration Record (MAR) charting system, adding a trigger to document the effects of pain medication. However, the trigger did not improve documentation for pain reassessment, perhaps because the MAR was computer-based and the Patient Care Flowsheet was in the bedside paper chart.

Unit leaders recognized that greater involvement in the data collection process would help achieve better overall pain assessment and management. Routine chart audits were selected as an appropriate solution.

FIGURE 3.
Unit Profile: 4East/4South

Overview   4East/4South is an acute care pediatric surgical trauma unit.

Unit	Staffed Beds	Total NHPPD	Hours Supplied by RNs (%)	RNs with BSN Degree (%)	RNs with National Certification (%)	Average RN Experience (years)
4East/4South	46	7.2	78	92	33	7

Note: NHPPD = Nursing hours per patient day.

NDNQI Case Studies in Nursing Quality Improvement

In 2006, the unit had successfully resolved an issue with under-medicating for pain through audits of the MAR and subsequent group discussions of patient scenarios combined with one-on-one coaching. Now, 4East/4South conducts monthly pain documentation audits to supplement the quarterly data obtained through participation in NDNQI.

Audits were designed to include a 24-hour assessment of pain management for all patients on the unit, focusing on reassessment since that was the unit's weakest point for compliance with the pain standard. Audits allowed timely feedback with bedside RNs. One-on-one coaching conversations at the point of care with peer auditors promoted resolution of problems in the AIR cycle, as well as prompt identification of pain management education needs. Collective audit results were distributed to all RNs via email and results were published in the unit newsletter.

As the audit initiative progressed, it was incorporated in nurses' performance evaluations and the unit's mission. A goal was set during staff evaluations: "Six months from this evaluation date, I will have consistently documented pain assessment scores on the flowsheet for initial assessment and reassessment post-intervention." Unit leaders were notified of any repeated noncompliance observed during audits. A mission statement was established for 4East/4South nurses to become experts in pain management. Specific objectives included improvement of pain assessment and reassessment documentation to 100% within 6 months.

Administrative Support

A team leader for this initiative was given four hours every month devoted to completing the audit, follow-up with staff, and any education planning. More time was allotted if requested. This cost approximately $160 per month. The team leader has a core group of staff who help with audits. As deemed necessary by the team leader, staff could be given four hours of dedicated time as well. Staff involvement and devoted time away from patient care allowed immediate follow-up

and planning when any issues were uncovered. This proved to be the most effective method to promoting consistent documentation behaviors.

Roll-out and Communication

Initially staff were told of the audit initiative in many forums, including staff meetings, nursing bedside rounds, emails, and pain management in-services. Once chart audits began, verbal announcements of scores were presented intermittently to staff. In-services educated staff about changes in flowsheet documentation, pain standards, and use of appropriate pain scales. Post tests were administered to evaluate learners' retention and understanding. A subcommittee of the unit's QPPS Council was formed to assist in the pain management re-education plan.

Monitoring Progress

The unit's NDNQI pain indicators and monthly chart audit scores have trended higher. In 2006 and 2007, NDNQI reports showed the unit's average number of pain assessments per patient per day was between 6.7 and 9.8. By the fourth quarter of 2008 and throughout 2009, this number ranged from 10.2 to 12.5 (see Figure 4). Thus, the unit's improvement efforts have increased the average number of pain assessments such that pain is now assessed almost every 2 hours around the clock. Equally important, the unit's average completion of AIR cycles was 96.6% in 2009, up from an average of 85.7% in 2006.

In addition to improvements in pain assessment and reassessment as a result of monthly chart audits and use of the hospital's new flowsheet, ongoing processes have been implemented to promote effective pain relief for patients on the unit. Each shift handoff includes a review of the patient's pain score and interventions used. Nursing rounds led by the clinical nurse specialist and weekly interprofessional rounds provide a forum to address any difficulties or concerns with current pain management and to formulate specific care plans as

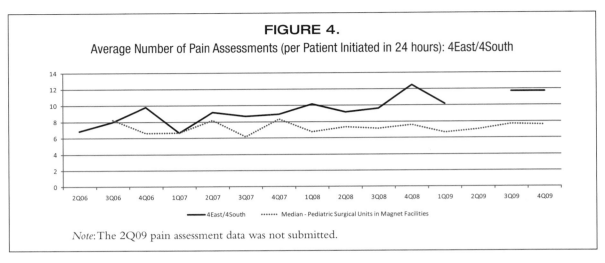

FIGURE 4.

Average Number of Pain Assessments (per Patient Initiated in 24 hours): 4East/4South

Legend: ——4East/4South ⋯⋯⋯ Median - Pediatric Surgical Units in Magnet Facilities

Note: The 2Q09 pain assessment data was not submitted.

needed, such as pain control during complex dressing changes. The hospital's Pain Management Service rounds twice each day. If a common theme or educational need is noted, the Service alerts unit leadership and discusses a plan for improvement. Pain nurse practitioners provide educational in-services quarterly on a wide variety of pain assessment and intervention topics.

Coaching conversations, either individually or with small groups, have been the most effective strategy in improving pain assessment and reassessment. Real-time feedback from peer auditors is especially valuable because of the immediate and specific discussions that occur and the timely changes that can be implemented. The unit's work to improve consistency in practice continues with more face-to-face positive feedback being provided for good documentation and pain management.

Unit-Specific Improvement Initiatives: 7West

Identification of the Problem and Potential Causes

During evaluation of quarterly NDNQI data, the unit's problem with documentation of pain assessments and reassessments became apparent. In 2006–2007, the average number of pain assessments was typically below the NDNQI mean for academic medical centers, and complete AIR cycles fell below 90%. The

7West QPPS representative informed 7West unit leaders about the barriers that nurses from other units had identified as potentially affecting pain assessment data. The 7West nurses agreed that potential causes such as lack of education about standards of pain management and disjointed, duplicate charting locations were problems on their unit, similar to barriers experienced by other CHOP units. In addition, 7West nurses realized the need for a pain assessment tool appropriate for the unit's neurologically impaired patient population. In response, the unit's QPPS representative participated in the nursing department's efforts to modify the documentation flowsheet while unit leaders set out to improve staff education about pain management and identify a nurse champion who would receive advanced training in pain assessment and management by joining the PRN group. (See Figure 5.)

Implementation of the Improvement Plan

A staff nurse was appointed as a unit-based pain resource nurse to serve as a liaison between 7West and the hospital's QPPS PRN subcommittee. The unit-based PRN was charged with educating her nursing colleagues about pain management and providing monthly updates about the PRN group's activities. The unit manager fully supported the unit PRN by providing paid time to attend hospital-wide PRN meetings and to prepare Lunch & Learn events, as well as covering costs of educational supplies. A member of

FIGURE 5.

FIGURE 5.

Unit Profile: 7West

Overview   7West is an acute care neurology and general pediatrics unit.

Unit	Staffed Beds	Total NHPPD	Hours Supplied by RNs (%)	RNs with BSN Degree (%)	RNs with National Certification (%)	Average RN Experience (years)
7West	25	8.9	73	93.5	9	4.2

Note: NHPPD = Nursing hours per patient day.

7West's leadership team attended a pain management conference in March 2008 to gain knowledge to assist the unit PRN with staff education.

The unit PRN brought successful strategies she had learned through involvement with the PRN group to 7West, such as monthly pain management audits. The unit PRN examined flowsheets for all patients admitted more than 24 hours before the audit. When documentation was not complete and correct, staff received direct feedback. This proved to be an effective strategy to modify staff behavior because it was done at the point of care and was conducted as a "teaching moment" rather than a disciplinary encounter.

When the unit PRN saw some decrease over time in the monthly audit results, she decided to initiate a new approach, measuring staff knowledge and beliefs about pediatric pain management to uncover barriers to practice. The staff were surveyed in August 2009 using the *Pediatric Nurses' Knowledge and Attitudes Survey* (City of Hope, 2002). Items with lower scores were used to create educational materials for Lunch & Learn presentations. For example, the unit PRN offered a Lunch & Learn presentation about developmentally appropriate pain assessment and management techniques with emphasis on teaching pain coping strategies. Case studies were used to provide concrete examples and facilitate discussion. A crossword puzzle was created to evaluate staff learning.

In October 2009, the rFLACC pain scale was rolled out hospital-wide. All 7West staff were educated one-on-one by the unit PRN. Use of the new tool was reinforced during monthly unit QPPS Council meetings. The rFLACC scale was especially relevant to nurses on 7West because they frequently care for children with neurological impairment or developmental delay. To evaluate use of this scale, the unit PRN conducted an audit of pain assessment tool selection. Weekly review of the unit census with attention to patients appropriate for the rFLACC scale was conducted. If the rFLACC scale had not been initiated within 24 hours of admission for an appropriate child, the PRN discussed this with staff to determine the barrier to use. As audits continued over time staff became aware of how useful the rFLACC scale was for the designated population, as it includes a discussion with the parent or guardian of the child regarding that child's usual pain behaviors.

Evaluating Progress

In 2007, 2008, and the first two quarters of 2009, the average number of pain assessments in 24 hours was between 3.4 and 5.7, with one exception in the first quarter of 2008. The third and fourth quarters of 2009 saw a rise to 6.3 and 8.2 (see Figure 6), due in part to the addition of the use of the rFLACC scale. The percent of complete AIR cycles rose as well, to an eight-quarter average of 98.2%.

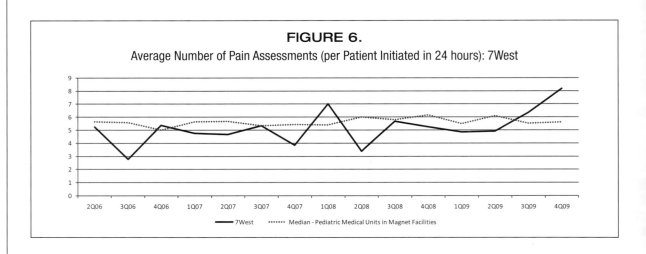

FIGURE 6.

Average Number of Pain Assessments (per Patient Initiated in 24 hours): 7West

—— 7West ⋯⋯⋯ Median - Pediatric Medical Units in Magnet Facilities

Multilevel Efforts Yielded Quality Gains

The PRN program and the pain assessment and documentation improvements instituted by the hospital's QPPS Council were well complemented by the monthly chart audits and ongoing individual and group peer education conducted by unit-based PRNs. Together these hospital-wide and unit-level efforts led to more frequent pain assessments and improved completion of AIR cycles. Ultimately, the improvements in assessment and reassessment translate into improved pain relief for pediatric patients.

References

All URLs were retrieved on December 10, 2010.

City of Hope Pain Resource Center. (2002). *Pediatric nurses' knowledge and attitudes survey.* http://prc.coh.org/pdf/PNKAS-2002.pdf

Hunt, A., Goldman, A., Seers, K., Crichton, N., Mastroyannopoulou, K., Moffat, V. et al. (2004). Clinical validation of the Paediatric Pain Profile. *Developmental Medicine & Child Neurology, 46*(1), 9–18.

Hunt, A., Wisbeach, A., Seers, K., Goldman, A., Crichton, N., Perry, L., & Mastroyannopoulou, K. (2007). Development of the Paediatric Pain Profile: Role of video analysis and saliva cortisol in validating a tool to assess pain in children with severe neurological disability. *Journal of Pain and Symptom Management, 33*(3), 276–289.

Malviya, S., Voepel-Lewis, T., Burke, C., Merkel, S., & Tait, A. R. (2006). The revised FLACC observational pain tool: Improved reliability and validity for pain assessment in children with cognitive impairment. *Pediatric Anesthesia, 16*(3), 258–265.

Voepel-Lewis, T., Malviya, S., & Tait, A. R. (2005). Validity of parent ratings as proxy measures of pain in children with cognitive impairment. *Pain Management Nursing, 6*(4), 168–174.

Voepel-Lewis, T., Merkel, S., Tait, A. R., Trzcinka, A., & Malviya, S. (2002). The reliability and validity of the face, legs, activity, cry, consolability observational tool as a measure of pain in children with cognitive impairment. *Anesthesia & Analgesia, 95*(5), 1224–1229.

Improving Pain Assessment and Management on Pediatric Medical-Surgical Units

Kimberly Eiden, APRN, MS, PCNS-BC
Clinical Nurse Specialist, Pediatric Pain Service
kimberly.eiden@advocatehealth.com

Advocate Hope Children's Hospital
Oak Lawn, Illinois
www.advocatehealth.com/hope

Case Study Highlights

The interprofessional Pediatric Pain and Comfort Team conducted a thorough baseline assessment of staff knowledge and patients' and parents' satisfaction with pain management, and then addressed the discovered gaps in performance (e.g., standardized age-appropriate assessments, revised pain treatment guidelines, expanded child life therapy services). The pediatric pain advanced practice nurse (APN) hired to lead the pain management program instituted more frequent audits of pain assessment and developed staff education based on audit results.

Identifying the Problem and Exploring Causes

According to the American Academy of Pediatrics (AAP) and the American Pain Society (APS), a substantial percentage of children are undertreated for acute and chronic pain, despite extensive literature that describes how to evaluate and treat pain in children. Personal values and beliefs of healthcare professionals about the meaning and value of pain in the development of a child (for instance, the belief that pain builds character) and about the treatment of pain cannot stand in the way of the optimal recognition and treatment of pain for all children (AAP & APS, 2001). As indicated by the experience of the Wisconsin Pain Initiative, a leading organization in the field of pain management endorsed by the Joint Commission, the establishment of an interprofessional workgroup is the first step in an organization's commitment to pain management (Gordon, Dahl, & Stevenson, 2000).

In 2005, Advocate Hope Children's Hospital (see Figure 1) established the Pediatric Pain and Comfort Team. The team recognized the necessity of conducting an institutional needs assessment as its first step in improving pain management. Baseline data were collected from multiple sources:

- A survey of staff knowledge and perceptions designed by the team and distributed to physicians, nurses, pharmacists, child life therapists, and ancillary staff.

- A survey of patients' and parents' satisfaction with pain management designed by the team.

- Post-discharge data from the Patient Satisfaction Survey question, "How well was your pain controlled?"

FIGURE 1.
Facility Profile

Advocate Hope Children's Hospital
Oak Lawn, Illinois
www.advocatehealth.com/hope

Facility overview	Advocate Hope Children's Hospital is a 69-bed children's specialty hospital that provides medical expertise in a child-centered environment. Advocate Hope Children's Hospital has participated in NDNQI since 2003.
Teaching status	Teaching
Ownership status	Not-for-profit
Magnet® status	Magnet-designated since 2005
Staffed beds	70
Affiliations	Advocate Christ Medical Center
Awards	Quint Studer Fire Starter Award, August 2009

Results from the survey of more than 300 staff demonstrated need for improvement in several areas, including standardized assessment and documentation, familiarity with policies and procedures related to pain, and more frequent use of child life therapy services. Child life therapists provide comfort, relaxation, and distraction during painful procedures and provide emotional support and education to patients and parents.

Data from patients and parents also demonstrated need for improvement. On the hospital's medical–surgical units (2 Hope and 4 Hope; see Figure 2), the post-discharge satisfaction with pain control scores were below the hospital's mean in 13 of 21 reporting periods. Of the patients and parents who responded to the Pediatric Pain and Comfort Team's survey, 28% responded that no pain rating scale was used to assess pain. Although many of the responses indicated that staff members asked about pain, no standardized tool was used for assessment and reassessment.

Pain Assessment and Management Improvement Initiatives

The Pediatric Pain and Comfort Team began to address the problems identified in the baseline data. Policies and guidelines needed to be developed to accomplish

FIGURE 2.
Unit Profiles

Overview This case study highlights improvements on two pediatric medical–surgical units.

Unit	Specialty	Staffed Beds	Total NHPPD	Hours Supplied by RNs (%)	RNs with BSN Degree (%)	RNs with National Certification (%)	Average RN Experience (years)
2 Hope	Telemetry/ Rehabilitation	24	9.9	70	68	24	11
4 Hope	Hemetology/ Oncology	22	9.8	100	66	22	9.7

Note: NHPPD = Nursing hours per patient day.

NDNQI Case Studies in Nursing Quality Improvement

consistent pain assessment and treatment among *all* staff. Education was needed regarding pain assessment tools, interventions, and reassessments (AIR), parent involvement, and pharmacological and non-pharmacological treatment modalities, along with an increased utilization of child life therapists.

To evaluate the process of pain assessment, nursing units began reporting data for NDNQI® pediatric pain assessment indicators. A change in the culture began as nursing leadership emphasized the importance of pain assessment and documentation. Unit managers started asking patients and families about pain during rounds. Daily group huddles were conducted by the unit managers, advanced practice nurses, and the pain management nurse to reinforce the need for proper assessment and documentation. The pain management nurse held a nursing grand round focused on which pain assessment tools were appropriate for each age and developmental group. Documentation using developmentally appropriate assessment tools was also presented in required pediatric care classes. While assessments may have been done in the past, they were not always charted, and therefore were seen as not done. Unit managers began random chart audits, reviewing the results during staff meetings and daily huddles. The APNs would talk individually with those associates who did not complete a full AIR cycle. With persistence, positive reinforcement, and accountability, an increase was seen in the number of pain assessments and documentation of complete AIR cycles.

To improve pain management, the Pediatric Pain and Comfort Team created a pocket handbook of simple guidelines for pain control during diagnostic and therapeutic procedures. The guidelines for each procedure were broken down by age and included appropriate pharmacological and non-pharmacological interventions (e.g., holding, touching, distracting, rocking, auditory stimulation). A house-wide pain medication dosing card was revised and guidelines were written for adjunct pain control techniques (cold sprays, pressure points, topical anesthetics, etc.). The creation and use of these tools led to a change in culture where nurses proactively treat for painful procedures.

Child life services were restructured so therapists would be assigned to units rather than by age groups. Child life therapists began assisting with all painful procedures, including blood draws and IV starts. The décor in treatment rooms was changed to provide distraction during procedures. Inpatient and emergency room staff received extensive re-education about strategies to decrease perception of pain during IV starts and blood draws and how to use the vein viewer. New procedural pain relief guide posters were developed and distributed throughout the hospital.

Following these initial steps, the team created a job description for a pediatric pain advanced practice nurse. This position was approved and recruited in early 2009. A memo was distributed to staff announcing the new role of the pediatric pain APN (May 2009) and a meet and greet was scheduled during staff meetings. The pediatric pain APN now coordinates the overall pain management program, collaborates with unit managers and unit-based APNs in identifying knowledge gaps, serves as a resource to both nursing and medical staff, and facilitates the pediatric pain quality measures.

The pediatric pain APN instituted more regular chart audits to ensure ongoing proper assessment and documentation. New education tools were based on the results of chart audits. Flyers are posted in the break rooms showing correct charting and documentation of pain. Pain assessment and management are also discussed in new RN orientation classes, in pediatric nursing grand rounds, and during in-services.

Administrative Support and Costs

Administrative support for improved pain management included establishing the full-time pediatric pain APN position, a new child life therapy position to cover the imaging department and emergency room, and a new part-time clinical practice partner, totaling $180,200 in annual salaries. The clinical practice partner was an RN completing her master's degree in order to advance to the role of Advanced Practice Nurse for the Pain Service. No cost to the hospital was incurred from

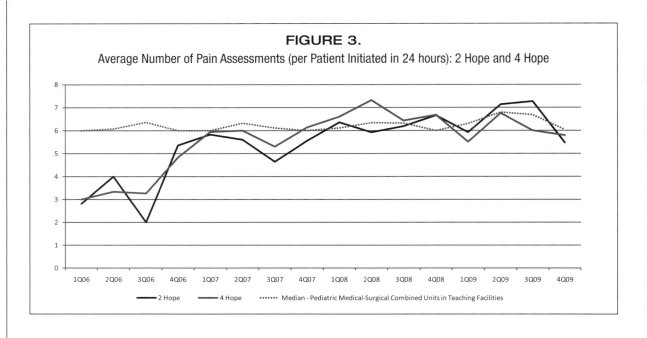

FIGURE 3.

Average Number of Pain Assessments (per Patient Initiated in 24 hours): 2 Hope and 4 Hope

2 Hope ——— 4 Hope ——— •••••• Median - Pediatric Medical-Surgical Combined Units in Teaching Facilities

increasing the number of pain assessments and improving documentation, as nurses were already conducting frequent patient rounds.

Monitoring Progress and Celebrating Success

The average number of pain assessments per patient in 24 hours has increased dramatically on 2 Hope and 4 Hope. In 2006, patients were only assessed two to four times per day. By 2008, patients were assessed approximately six times per day (see Figure 3), near the NDNQI median for pediatric medical–surgical units in teaching hospitals. Most importantly, the frequency of pain assessment now matches the hospital's nursing policy. In 2008 and 2009, 2 Hope and 4 Hope both achieved 100% completion of AIR cycles in 7 out of 8 quarters, for an 8-quarter average of 99.6% and 99.2%, respectively.

The hospital's post-discharge Patient Satisfaction Survey scores also rose substantially. Hospital-wide, satisfaction with pain control increased from the 33rd percentile in 2007 to the 85th percentile in 2009. For the medical–surgical units specifically, 2 Hope had scored at the 50th percentile and 4 Hope had scored

at the 76th percentile in 2007. In 2009, 2 Hope scored at the 86th percentile while 4 Hope scored at the 95th percentile for satisfaction with pain control. To celebrate this increase in patient satisfaction scores, a staff *thank you* luncheon was provided by the pediatric leadership team.

Ongoing Efforts to Maintain Success

Improved pain assessment and management has been a gradual change. Advocate Hope Children's Hospital has transformed its culture to one that continuously assesses for and treats patients in pain. By doing so, dramatic improvement in NDNQI pain indicators and patient satisfaction scores have been achieved. However, the work is not over. The hospital will continuously look for ways to improve scores and strive for 100% AIR cycle fulfillment on all units, all the time. Care processes continue to be revised as needed (the hospital recently pilot tested new guidelines for relief of pain related to vaso-occlusive crisis in patients with sickle cell). In October 2010, the hospital hosted a Pediatric Pain Symposium to provide further education about effective pain management. These ongoing efforts will help maintain and advance the successful improvement of pain assessment and treatment.

References

American Academy of Pediatrics & American Pain Society (AAP & APS). (2001). The assessment and management of acute pain in infants, children, and adolescents. *Pediatrics, 108*(3), 793–797.

Gordon, D., Dahl, J. L., & Stevenson, K. K. (2000). *Building an institutional commitment to pain management: The Wisconsin resource manual* (2nd ed.). Madison, WI: University of Wisconsin-Madison Board of Regents.

Chapter 4.
Lessons Learned and the Future of Nursing Quality

Improvements in nursing quality result from evidence-based changes in the structure and processes of care. From unit-specific to system-wide initiatives, in hospitals of various types and sizes, the case studies in Chapter 3 demonstrate the teamwork and persistent effort required to achieve better patient outcomes. This chapter summarizes some of the lessons that can be drawn from the case studies and discusses future directions in nursing quality improvement.

Structural improvements were a hallmark of these case studies. Hospitals hired new staff, especially nurses with advanced specialty training who provided expertise and mentoring for direct-care nurses. Resource nurse programs trained staff nurses as experts for their peers. Getting specialized knowledge to the bedside was a central theme in structural improvement. Depending on the factors contributing to each problem, units were reorganized, nurse–patient ratios were improved, the percent of hours supplied by agency staff was reduced, and nursing skill mix was optimized. Hospitals also purchased new equipment. By providing nurses with the supplies needed to give evidence-based quality care, negative outcomes such as pressure ulcers, falls, and infections were reduced. The costs of new equipment and salaries for additional staff were more than recouped by the savings from fewer adverse events.

Hospitals and units also instituted process improvements, especially more frequent data collection and immediate post-event analysis. Monthly prevalence studies and chart audits were used to identify and correct factors contributing to pressure ulcers or inadequate pain assessment. Similarly, weekly meetings and same-day post-fall reviews allowed leaders and bedside nurses to quickly correct deficiencies and recognize prevention needs. Frequent monitoring and direct one-on-one coaching by peers and leaders promoted cultures of accountability and led to further ideas for improvement.

Other care processes were revised as well. Daily rounds were commonly used to bring increased attention to skin care issues and promote frequent review of device necessity. QI teams designed new prevention protocols based on research literature. Importantly, risk categories were matched to specific interventions. Targeting the right patients with the right techniques not only improves outcomes but uses nursing time and resources efficiently. Daily shift huddles promoted communication and teamwork. New documentation forms streamlined nurses' work. The process changes used in the case studies brought practice in line with current scientific knowledge and addressed the core issues behind each quality problem.

All of these changes were designed and implemented by teams. Often interprofessional and indicator-specific, the teams were frequently part of a larger quality council empowered by hospital administrators to make the changes needed to improve care. Teams rolled out new procedures using a variety of means, such as online education, in-services, posters, emails, pocket handbooks, and staff meetings. To sustain motivation for improvement, hospitals used real-time feedback on incident-free days and rewarded staff when milestones were reached.

Beyond the specific techniques that hospitals used to reform the structure and processes of care, these case studies demonstrate the effort and persistence required to achieve real improvement. Multiple strategies, dedicated teams and staff, and years of effort are involved. Often, original plans were revised and expanded in order to reach improvement goals. As Berwick, Godfrey, & Roessner (1990) aptly noted, "Quality improvement in health care is not a static fixture; it is a lifelong endeavor. What we try today, we will change tomorrow. We will improve improvement itself as we learn and grow together."

Indeed, nursing quality improvement continues to advance in new directions. The typical nursing work environment is characterized by inefficiencies and distractions like searching for supplies or being interrupted during patient care tasks (Tucker & Spear, 2006). Nurse researchers are studying distractions in an effort to make nursing units safer and more efficient (Brixey, Robinson, Turlye, & Zhang, 2010; Ebright, Patterson, Chalko, & Render, 2003; Potter, Wolf, Boxerman, Grayson, Sledge et al., 2005). Redesigned work environments will cut non-value-added RN activities to give nurses more time at the bedside (Institute of Medicine, 2010). In the future, these new evidence-based structural changes will be widely implemented and result in better patient outcomes.

In addition to existing quality indicators, new nursing-sensitive indicators will be used in the future. The role of nurses in reducing readmissions, issues surrounding patient hand-offs, and outcomes in specialty practice areas are all ripe for indicator development. The scope of pain management indicators may be expanded as well. The future will also bring an emphasis on measuring the processes that support positive patient outcomes.

NDNQI will continue to be a leader in nursing quality measurement. As nursing-sensitive indicators are increasingly integrated into public reporting and pay-for-performance, the value of the nursing profession grows. Dedicated to excellent care, nurses will continue to use data from their practice to advocate for patient safety and improved quality.

References

All URLs were retrieved on December 10, 2010.

Berwick, D. M., Godfrey, A. B., & Roessner, J. (1990). *Curing health care: New strategies for quality improvement.* San Francisco, CA: Jossey-Bass.

Brixey, J. J., Robinson, D. J., Turley, J. P., & Zhang, J. (2010). The roles of MDs and RNs and initiators and recipients of interruptions in workflow. *International Journal of Medical Informatics, 79*(6), 109–115.

Ebright, P. R., Patterson, E. S., Chalko, B. A., & Render, M. L. (2003). Understanding the complexity of registered nurse work in acute care settings. *Journal of Nursing Administration, 33*(12), 630–638.

Institute of Medicine (IOM). (2010). Quality and safety: Improving care through nurse empowerment. In *A Summary of the October 2009 Forum on the Future of Nursing: Acute Care* (Chap. 3). http://www.nap.edu/openbook .php?record_id=12855&page=15

Potter, P., Wolf, L., Boxerman, S., Grayson, D., Sledge, J., Dunagan, C., & Evanoff, B. (2005). Understanding the cognitive work of nursing in the acute care environment. *Journal of Nursing Administration, 35*(7–8), 327–335.

Tucker, A. L., & Spear, S. J. (2006). Operational failures and interruptions in hospital nursing. *Health Services Research, 41*(3 Pt. 1), 643–662.

Appendix A.
NDNQI Measures by Category

NDNQI® collects the following nursing-sensitive indicators each quarter of the calendar year, with the exception of nursing work environment indicators, which are collected through an annual survey of RNs. (The survey is comprised of structure measures, process measures, nurse outcomes, and patient outcomes.) All indicators are reported by unit type with comparison data from peer hospitals.

Indicators that are National Quality Forum (NQF) Consensus Standards are marked with an asterisk (*).

Structure of Nursing Care Measures

Nursing Care Hours
- Total nursing hours per patient day*
- Registered nurse (RN) hours per patient day*

Skill Mix
- Percent of total nursing hours supplied by:
  —RNs*
  —Licensed practical nurses (LPNs) and/or licensed vocational nurses (LVNs)*
  —Unlicensed assistive personnel*
  —Agency staff*

RN Education and Certification
- Percent of RNs with BSN or higher nursing degree
- Percent of RNs with national certification

Nurse Turnover
- Total turnover rates (percent of staff who separate and percent of FTEs [full-time employees] lost for any reason)
- Voluntary turnover rate (percent of staff who separate voluntarily; adapted from NQF for unit-level data)*
- Magnet®-controllable turnover rate (percent of FTEs lost for Magnet-controllable reasons)

Nursing Work Environment
- Practice Environment Scale*
- Index of Work Satisfaction (adapted for unit-level data)
- Nursing Work Index (adapted for unit-level data)
- Job Enjoyment Scale
- Work Context (e.g., floating, meal breaks, overtime, etc.)

Processes of Nursing Care Measures

Pressure Ulcer Prevention
- Percent of all patients with a risk assessment (on admission and within past 24 hours)
- Percent of at-risk patients receiving:
  —Skin assessment
  —Pressure-reducing surface
  —Repositioning
  —Nutritional support
  —Moisture management

Fall Prevention
- Percent of all patients with a risk assessment (on admission and within last 24 hours)
- Percent of at-risk patients on a fall prevention protocol
- Percent of patients with restraints in use when they fell

Pediatric Pain Assessment

- Average number of pain assessments per patient initiated in 24 hours

- Percent of completed pain assessment-intervention-reassessment (AIR) cycles

Patient Outcomes Measures

Pressure Ulcers

- Percent of surveyed patients with hospital-acquired pressure ulcers

- Percent of surveyed patients with hospital-acquired pressure ulcers Stage II or greater★

- Percent of surveyed patients with unit-acquired pressure ulcers

Patient Falls

- Total falls per 1,000 patient days★

- Injury falls per 1,000 patient days★

- Percent of all falls that resulted in moderate or greater injury

Healthcare-Associated Infections

- Central line-associated blood stream infections per 1,000 central line days★

- Catheter-associated urinary tract infections per 1,000 catheter days★

- Ventilator-associated pneumonia per 1,000 ventilator days★

Restraint Prevalence

- Percent of patients in physical restraints (limb and/or vest)★

Psychiatric Physical/Sexual Assault Rate

- Total assaults per 1,000 patient days

- Injury assaults per 1,000 patient days

Pediatric Peripheral IV (PIV) Infiltration

- Percent of PIV sites with infiltrations

Appendix B.
Resources for Quality Improvement

In addition to NDNQI® reports, additional sources of information will be needed by nurses undertaking quality improvement activities, including information on quality improvement, evidence-based practice guidelines, and organizational change theory and practice. The following list of resources will provide readers with a starting point for gathering such corollary information. The list is by no means exhaustive, but provides many of the most widely used sources.

All URLs were retrieved December 10, 2010.

Tools and Resources for Quality Improvement

Agency for Healthcare Research and Quality (AHRQ) Health Care Innovations Exchange
http://www.innovations.ahrq.gov/

American Society for Quality (ASQ) Quality in Healthcare
http://www.asq.org/healthcare-use/why-quality/overview.html

Institute for Healthcare Improvement (IHI) Improvement Map
http://www.ihi.org/IHI/Programs/ImprovementMap/

Interdisciplinary Nursing Quality Research Initiative
http://www.inqri.org/

Interpreting and Using Your NDNQI Reports
Interactive online training to help NDNQI hospitals understand and use their NDNQI reports. (Log in to https://www.nursingquality.org/, then select Learning Center from the main menu.)

Joint Commission Patient Safety Initiatives
http://www.jointcommission.org/PatientSafety/

National Association of Healthcare Quality (NAHQ)
http://www.nahq.org/

Patient Safety and Quality: An Evidence-Based Handbook for Nurses
http://www.ahrq.gov/QUAL/nurseshdbk/

Guidelines and Intervention Bundles

Association for Professionals in Infection Control and Epidemiology (APIC): Elimination Guides
http://www.apic.org/Content/NavigationMenu/PracticeGuidance/APICEliminationGuides/APIC_Elimination_Gui.htm

Healthcare-Associated Infection Prevention Compendium
http://www.cdc.gov/ncidod/dhqp/HAI_shea_idsa.html

Infectious Disease Society of America (IDSA): Practice Guidelines
http://www.idsociety.org/Content.aspx?id= 9088

Institute for Healthcare Improvement (IHI) Bundles
http://www.ihi.org/IHI/Topics/CriticalCare/IntensiveCare/ImprovementStories/WhatIsaBundle.htm

National Guidelines Clearinghouse
http://www.guideline.gov/

National Pressure Ulcer Advisory Panel (NPUAP): Pressure Ulcer Prevention
http://www.npuap.org/Final_Quick_Prevention_for_web_2010.pdf

Veterans Affairs National Center for Patient Safety (NCPS): Fall Prevention and Management
http://www.patientsafety.gov/CogAids/FallPrevention/index.html#page=page-1

Other Organizational Resources

Agency for Healthcare Research and Quality (AHRQ):

Mistake-Proofing the Design of Health Care Processes
http://www.ahrq.gov/qual/mistakeproof/
mistakeproofing.pdf

Centers for Medicare and Medicaid Services (CMS):

Quality Initiatives: General Information
https://www.cms.gov/QualityInitiativesGenInfo/01_
overview.asp

National Association for Healthcare Quality (NAHQ):

Journal for Healthcare Quality
http://www.nahq.org

National Quality Forum (NQF):

*Measurement Framework: Evaluating Efficiency Across
Patient-Focused Episodes of Care*
http://www.qualityforum.org/Publications/2010/01/
Measurement_Framework__Evaluating_Efficiency_
Across_Patient-Focused_Episodes_of_Care.aspx

Safe Practices for Better Healthcare: 2010 Update
http://www.qualityforum.org/Publications/2010/04/
Safe_Practices_for_Better_Healthcare_–_2010_Update
.aspx

Quality and Safety Education for Nurses (QSEN):
http://www.qsen.org/

Articles, Magazines, and Books

Berwick, D. M., Godfrey, A. B., & Roessner, J. (1990). *Curing health care: New strategies for quality improvement.* San Francisco, CA: Jossey-Bass.

Dunton, N., Gajewski, B., Taunton, R. L., Moore, J. (2004). Nurse staffing and patient falls on acute care hospital units. *Nursing Outlook, 52* (1), 53–59.

Dunton, N., & Montalvo, I. (2009). *Sustained improvement in nursing quality: Hospital performance on NDNQI indicators, 2007–2008.* Silver Spring, MD: Nursesbooks.org.

Finkelman, A., & Kenner, C. (2009). *Teaching IOM: Implications of the Institute of Medicine reports for nursing education* (2nd ed.). Silver Spring, MD: Nursesbooks.org.

Graban, M. (2009). *Lean hospitals: Improving quality, patient safety, and employee satisfaction.* Boca Raton, FL: CRC Press. (See also associated web site: http://www.lean-hospitalsbook.com/)

Harris, R. L. (1999). *Information graphics: A comprehensive illustrated reference.* New York, NY: Oxford University Press.

Heath, C., & Heath, D. (2010). *Switch: How to change things when change is hard.* New York, NY: Crown Publishing Group, Random House, Inc. (See also associated web site: http://heathbrothers.com/switch/)

Institute of Medicine (IOM). (2001). *Crossing the quality chasm: A new health system for the 21st century.* Washington, DC: National Academies Press. http://www.nap.edu/catalog.php?record_id=10027

Langley, G. J., Moen, R. D., Nolan, K. M., Nolan, T. W., Norman, C. L., & Provost, L. P. (2009). *The improvement guide: A practical approach to enhancing organizational performance* (2nd ed.). San Francisco, CA: Jossey-Bass.

Montalvo, I., & Dunton, N. (2007). *Transforming nursing data into quality care: Profiles of quality improvement in U.S. healthcare facilities.* Silver Spring, MD: Nursesbooks.org.

Patient Safety and Quality Healthcare Magazine, http://www.psqh.com/index.php

Index

**NDNQI Case Studies in
Nursing Quality Improvement**

quality improvement (*continued*)

    evidence-based structures and processes, 12, 14, 15–16

    goal setting, 11–12

    identifying areas for, 9, 12–14

    implementing, 16–18

    recognizing success, 19

    staffing and structural improvements critical, 99

    steps in, 9f

    tools and resources for, 103–104

    See also NDNQI reports in quality improvement

quality indicators, 1, 2, 3, 4f

    for evaluating nursing care, 3–5

    structure, process, and outcomes indicators, 3–5, 4f

R

reimbursement, 1, 3, 55

restraint prevalence measures (NDNQI), 102

RN education and certification measure (NDNQI), 101

root cause analysis, 6, 12–13

    in case studies, 16, 49, 51, 75, 81, 82

S

safety issues, 1–2, 55, 71, 71f, 73

Scripps Memorial Hospital case study, 47–53

    See also hospital-acquired pressure ulcers

sexual assault rate measures (NDNQI), 102

Shands Hospital, case study, 23–30

    See also hospital-acquired pressure ulcers

skill mix measures, 101

skin assessment and care issues, 16–17, 36f, 42, 50–52

    See also hospital-acquired pressure ulcers

St. John Medical Center case study, 31–37

    See also hospital-acquired pressure ulcers

St. Luke's Episcopal Hospital case study, 69–74

    See also patient falls

staff training in quality improvement, 29, 41, 42, 77, 90, 91

staffing issues, 5, 13, 51, 52, 65, 95, 99

structural factors and quality of care, 14–15, 99

    organizational issues, 5–6, 63

    in quality improvement, 48–49

structure indicators in evaluating nursing care, 3–5, 4f

W

Washington Hospital Center case study, 16, 39–45

    See also hospital-acquired pressure ulcers

WOCN. *See* wound, ostomy, and continence nurses

workplace culture and work environment in quality improvement, 6, 15, 48–52

    NDNQI measures of, 101

wound, ostomy, and continence nurses and HAPU reduction, 39, 41, 42

    case study, 23–30

    program success factors, 26–27

    resource nurse model, 14, 25–26

    See also hospital-acquired pressure ulcers